LEAN HAPPY HEALTHY YOU
8 healthy habits for her happy life

Copyright 2016, 2019 by Michelle Bernard
All rights reserved.

The Live Above Ordinary Oasis

https://liveaboveordinary.teachable.com

Library of Congress Cataloging-in-Publication Data
Michelle Bernard
Lean Happy Healthy You revised 2nd edition
ISBN 9781797655390 soft cover

The author of this book does not prescribe the use of any technique
or exercise as a form of treatment for physical, emotional, or medical
problems without the advice of a physician or licensed therapist,
either directly or indirectly. The information therein is of a general
nature to help you in your quest for emotional, mental, and physical
well-being. The author assumes no responsibility for your actions.

Second Edition

Also from Michelle Bernard

beyond words—finding fulfillment between the lines

PAPER COACH, a wellness journal & log

WHATEVER | A JOURNAL FOR THE STUFF I THINK - for tweens & teens

the black coffee journal series including journaling cards

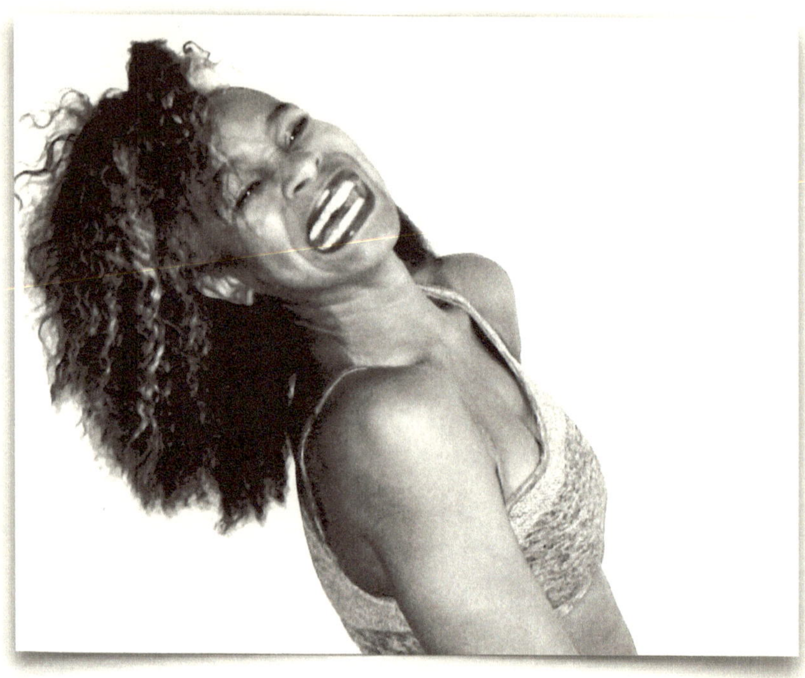

LEAN HAPPY HEALTHY YOU

8 healthy habits for her happy life

DISCLAIMER

Always consult your healthcare specialist for an individualized diagnosis and
treatment.
Never begin a fitness/nutrition program without your health specialist's
approval.

Factors such as medications, age, and intensity can affect the quality of
results.

◆

When addressing physical and mental health in any of our websites, videos,
audios, books, and/or programs, whether in-person, text, or via the internet,
we have taken every effort to ensure that we accurately represent our
programs and their ability to improve your wellness.
However, by purchasing any of our products, you accept and fully agree to
the responsibility to consult with your certified health-care specialist.
You, alone, are responsible for any personal omissions or additions to the
program, as directed by your licensed physician.
The information contained in our books, websites, and programs, whether in-
person, text, or via the internet cannot replace or substitute for services from
licensed medical professionals.
Our programs, coaching, products, partners, or affiliates' programs are not
created as a treatment to any illness.

You agree to use the author's suggestions, websites, products, and links at
your own risk.

Got it?
Super. Now let's elevate your life.

Elliot, Anna, Goss
You are my great teachers. Thank you.

M. Todd Bernard
Your relentless pursuit has fueled mine.

habit

a usual way of behaving

CONTENTS

LEAN HAPPY HEALTHY YOU

8 healthy habits for her happy life

A HAPPY RETURN	1
EVERYONE CAN LOSE WEIGHT	3
THE EYES HAVE IT	6
IS IT GONNA HURT?	8
FAMILIARITY AND FEAR ARE BOTH F-WORDS	11
THE BEST WAY TO USE THIS BOOK	15

PART ONE—IDENTITY — 20
I HATE EXERCISE	21
I HAVE NO IDEA HOW THE WEIGHT FELL OFF	34
WE'RE IN THE BEGINNING (WE CAN AIM FOR A HAPPY MIDDLE)	43
DECIDE	46

PART TWO—FOCUS — 48
THE CHARLIE BROWN SOLUTION	50
DECISION FATIGUE	51
ROUTINE REQUIRES LESS ENERGY	54
HABIT	57
POINT OF FOCUS	60

YOU'VE PROGRAMMED A SET OF BELIEFS ABOUT YOUR
BODY   61
THE PROGRAM   63
CHOOSE YOUR PRINCIPLES   69
WHAT'S POSSIBLE?   73
THE RITUAL   77
THE DUMP   79

PART THREE—LIVE   **83**
HEALTHY HABITS FOR YOUR MIND   85
HEALTHY HABITS FOR YOUR HEART   105
HEALTHY HABITS FOR YOUR BODY   129

PART FOUR—TRUST   **273**
BACK AWAY FROM THE SCALE   274
MEASURE YOUR PROGRESS   277
UNDRAPE YOUR MASTERPIECE   280
IS THIS YOU?   281
FIND A TRIBE THAT ALIGNS WITH YOUR VIBE   285
ALL YOU NEED IS...   289
MAKE PEACE WITH TIME   292
SQUIRREL!   296

PART FIVE—YOUR HAPPY PLACE   **304**
MAGIC LIGHT   307
THE HAPPY RETURN   309

ABOUT THE AUTHOR   315

Referenced Links

Referenced Books

Referenced Film

Estimate Your Heart Rate

UNBREAKABLE?   322

My FĀV Things

A HAPPY RETURN

Does any of this weight-loss stuff actually work?

For years you've dragged yourself to crack-of-dawn boot camps to hurt the fat away. You'd choke down a miracle fruit from middle earth if it would reduce your appetite. This year, you own two health club memberships and an expired class-card to Total-Fit. You've invested years of time and money to make that darn fat disappear, but no matter how hard you've tried, the weight remains happy at home—on your belly.

While straddling hope and aggravation, you doubt whether it's even possible to lose 20 pounds. No wonder you binged on pizza and cheese sticks at your niece's birthday party. You had to—there was nothing else to eat. Plus, everyone was eating it; you didn't want to be rude. And last night, after you rubbed the cellulite dissolvent over your hips, you treated yourself to a sugarless ice cream sandwich... well, two sugarless ice cream sandwiches. You had to—you deserve something more interesting than the celery leaf soup you slurped for dinner.

Ugh! is an understatement for your plight. Should you just give up on the whole thing and go back to scarfing down those doughnuts before work? Yeah, you've thought about it. Yet, you keep getting pulled back to *what if?*

What if I could wear a bikini on my next vacation to Punta Cana?
What if shopping for clothes wasn't such a downer?
What if I could show up at my high school reunion wearing the same dress size I wore in high school?
What if I could wake up excited, energized, and confident?
What if I could get through the day without feeling exhausted, old, and uninspired?

So far, you've gotten nowhere near a happy return for your investments, but you're not totally ready to jump off the "I give up" cliff.

Listen, my lady, you are about to receive your happy return for your investment. You're about to get the results you've intended.

You're much more than a body. You are a person with responsibilities and obligations to your work, family, and community. You have personal interests and aversions. You have acquired a treasure of experiences, memories and dreams during your lifetime. All of these things play a role in your weight-loss journey.

EVERYONE CAN LOSE WEIGHT

Even you.

If you start exercising today, three times a week for only 30 minutes each time, you will lose *some* weight—and you might even keep it off for a while. If you go on a diet, any diet written in any book you already have on your bookshelf or Kindle, you will lose weight. You already know this. Except this time, you want to keep the weight lost for good. You want results that move you forward, not backward or sideways.

The 8 habits in LEAN HAPPY HEALTHY YOU will progress you forward. You'll be able to lose excess fat, easily 5-10 pounds in the first 7 weeks, and gain lean muscle to shape your body and strengthen your bones. You'll learn how to choose foods that energize and support your daily activities. Perhaps those are the things you'd expect from a person with my title.

I'm a wellness and lifestyle consultant. I coach women of various ages and body-types to achieve their health goals using strength training, fitness, dance, yoga, and journaling. I utilize the universal fitness habits along with affirmative mental techniques. Both are necessary if you want long-term results. The 8 healthy practices in this book—I fondly call them *The RiTual*—are based on universal wellness practices and my personal experience spanning over twenty years. These habits would have expedited my initial transformation thirty years ago. Given that I was able to try-on so many *unsuccessful* ways of dropping pounds over the years, I can assure you I've selected 8 healthy habits that **will** transform your body.

During PART ONE, I'll share my weight-loss journey. Living as an over-eater seemed my destiny. I went from secretly hating my body to being able to express crazy-love for it.

In PART TWO, I'll show you how to direct your mind toward your goal. It's the only way you'll be able to change your body. During PART THREE and PART FOUR, you'll practice the 8 healthy habits of *The RiTual.* You'll also learn how to slip into pockets of ease and rejuvenation throughout your day. During PART FIVE, I'll

present the number one way for you to get your
happiest return of wellness.

Value yourself. Integrate the practices from this book into
your busy life without delay. Let your worth be reflected
by the choices you make every day. You can become
who you truly intend to be in every area of your life.
I support you.

Michelle Bernard, one happy lady

THE EYES HAVE IT

I've worked with so many women who want to reduce back-fat and shrink clapping thighs. If this is you, imagine your answer to this question.

How do you desire to look and feel one year from today?

Not a hard question, eh?
Okay, answer it—right now. I'll wait.

Did you imagine your answer, or did you shy away from the image that came to mind? If you backed out of your vision after the first 5 seconds, try again.

Right on. I have another question.

Do you believe the vision you've had of your body and life is possible in real-life?

The answers to those two questions will either unlock success for you or keep you far from it.

You have authority over your mind. You have authority over your fitness. You have the authority to improve your body's general state of health and the authority to elevate your self-concept. Begin by imagining exactly what you want.

Visualize your body in another way. For a moment forget about getting ripped abs (oh God, that's hard) or having strong, sculpted shoulders in your open-back dress (I'm biting my fist to do this).

Consider *the way* of your body—your health.

Do you think it's healthy to belch 46 times a day? Nah. Do you think it's healthy to suck down pink and green Tums to neutralize the clawing at your ribs? Is it common to nurse a low-grade headache that lasts all work week? Is the last hour at work cued by the belly bloat you feel every day?

Constipation, indigestion, rashes that won't go away, feeling bloated after 3 pm are uncomfortable signs that something's not right. I used to wonder if I was the only one who felt so bad when some of these discomforts became normalized for me. I hoped to rid myself of these aches with no idea how to change them.

These health issues do not have to plague you. Each of them can be 75-100% eradicated with a healthy lifestyle shift. You deserve to reap the benefits of living healthy.

IS IT GONNA HURT?

Is this process gonna hurt? Sometimes. You will bump into discomfort—sometimes.

You probably weren't expecting that answer.

I could cheer you along while hiding a sinister smile under my downward dog. I could do a cartwheel while singing *You have nothing to fear!* I could mislead you and say I've found a way to make fat-loss easier and faster than ever. That's what we'd all like to hear, especially because life's other responsibilities are hard enough to endure, right? Why would you want to choose **The RiTual** if might hurt at some point?

The process of losing weight and changing your body might hurt at times—but un-crinkle your forehead—the discomfort will only be temporary. The pain from **not** living healthy is an agony that will never end.

Here's why this healthy process might hurt temporarily.
Your body and mind are comfortable doing what feels
familiar, even if what's *familiar* has damaged your health
or bludgeoned your confidence. To be able to change
your body, you'll need to embody new habits that
eventually become your *new familiar way of being*. The
adjustment period might be uncomfortable.

Temporary discomfort has truncated many-an-effort to
lose body fat. "Discomfort" can sound like this:

I couldn't make it to my workout(s) today because...
- My yoga pants were dirty.
- It was raining.
- My boyfriend asked me to make his favorite lasagna
dish last night.
- My girlfriend and I rarely get to see each other so I
met her for a 5 drinks.
- I just got my hair done.
- I just got my toes done.
- I was sleepy.
- Time got away from me.

If any of these excuses have come out of your mouth,
then maintaining a consistent exercise program might
make you feel uncomfortable at first.

"Discomfort" breeds excuses that'll sabotage you from maintaining consistent workouts.

- I forgot to buy a lock.
- I need new sneakers.
- I have too many holiday parties this month.
- I'm too hungry.
- Someone called me right as I was leaving for the gym.
- I want to lose weight first. (Huh?)
- I'm too busy these days, so I'm gonna start working out again after the new year, after I finish finals, after I change jobs—when, after, before, if...

Arm-wrestle this cast of procrastination players, or you'll never unzip your duffle bag.

Has it been difficult for you to commit or follow-through with your fitness and health goal?
Are you afraid of the temporary discomfort?
Do you fear you'll miss out on something?

If your answers are YES, you might be one who'll raise excuses and delay your happy return. Be aware that you might be sore after your workouts. It might be hard to breathe, balance, or keep-up during certain types of exercise. But, your stamina and strength will improve if

you keep going. You might have to say "no" to the free
pizza at work. Keep going. Your palate will change, and
it will feel empowering to say "no" after a while.

Think of the physical discomfort you'll transcend because
of regular exercise and healthy eating like heartburn,
swollen ankles, acne breakouts, and the anxiety about
what you'll wear because nothing fits. It's so worth it,
right?

FAMILIARITY AND FEAR
ARE BOTH F-WORDS

Discomfort and pain might trigger your fears to surface.

*Will I have to trade in my regular way of life for a
tougher, boring, redundant life?*
Will I forever miss out on having fun with my friends?
*Will I never be able to eat a slice of my mama's peach
pie?*
*Will I spend hundreds of personal training bucks and
never reduce my gut?*
*Will I struggle for six months only to drop four measly
pounds?*

What are you afraid to experience during this transformation?

It's good for you to bring your answer to this question out from the dark. Look at it. Maybe it's a valid fear. Maybe it would never happen. Maybe it's too soon for you to consider such a fear, because the outcome might not be as intense as you've imagined.

Do you believe you're sentenced by genetics, so why bother? Genetics can influence your body's physical disposition or somatotype, but a healthy lifestyle can have up to a 75% effect over genetics.

I'll explain somatotypes in habit #5. Current research has proven that your body shape, weight, and health are impacted by your somatotype. However, your specific lifestyle and environment can drastically change your body and health. The newest research of epigenetics shows that your internal environment is just as influential as your external one. Your lifestyle choices including your thoughts, behaviors, the people you spend the most time with, and your long-held beliefs are large and in-charge of your body and health.

You will have to make changes to your daily mental and physical habits in order to lose weight. You'll need to be conscious about these changes so you don't slip back into an old, familiar, less-healthy lifestyle.

Discomfort is gonna take you by the hand when your Mother-in-law pushes the gargantuan slice of chocolate cake up to your nose after you've said *I'll have a small piece, please* three times. Discomfort will smush your cheeks into your teeth when you have to tell your Aunt Sue that you don't want to try her macaroni and cheese because the sweet potato on your plate is all the starch you want to eat for the meal. You might feel uncomfortable convincing yourself to forfeit 15 minutes of sleep in exchange for the boot camp Yoga class before work. Anytime you arrive at a fork in the road during your transformation, you'll meet two arrows that say *what I used to do* and *who I'm becoming now*. Choosing can feel uncomfortable.

There is a happy-ending, though. The decision to consciously erect a healthy lifestyle is going to take you where you intend to go—5-10 pounds of fat-loss in 7 weeks—so choose the *who I'm becoming now* arrow.

Guess what else could happen? After nine months living with new healthy habits, most of your discomfort will disappear. You'll feel energized, optimistic, and confident in your new body. You'll stand before mirrors grinning. You'll zip your dress without inhaling. You won't have to wear pants with an elastic waistband to Thanksgiving dinner.

By then, when your buddies shuffle their sucky-body comments like decks of cards, when they slap their complaints onto the table of conversation daring someone else to top 'em, you won't fold. You won't be able to relate. Your new lifestyle will have conquered your old complaints. A little discomfort is gonna take you to the life and body you've always wanted.

The best way to use this book

....

CAMP OUT WITH IT

....

This is probably not your first time at the rodeo. If you've read other books on exercise and health, some of this content won't seem new. However, the way you use this book might feel new. Camp out with it.

Your learning curve surges when you implement information right away. There's a curve for forgetting information, too. If the content in this book is not integrated right away, up to 80% of it will be forgotten— lost to the ethers, hitched to a puff of smoke. Gone, as if it never happened.

To benefit from these 8 habits, you gotta *put them on*.

Here's how to *put them on*:
1. Take notes. Record your takeaways.
2. Practice the habits right away.
3. Share **The RiTual**. Teach the habits to somebody else.

1. **Take notes.** You'll retain 50% more if you do. Detail your takeaways. Marry the material to your memory with your pen or stylus. When these habits become a part of your personal experience, you'll practice them with less mental effort.

I've helped with the *take notes* stuff. Sharpen your pencil or get your silky pen. There are places for you to CAMP OUT with the habits. At the end of each section there's a camp ground to stake your tent of notes.

In each camp ground you'll be prompted to CHECK IN and review the section. After that, CAMP OUT and PRACTICE THE HABIT.

Journaling questions are strewn throughout the book. Journaling lets you observe your personal habits and thoughts. Keep a **journal** while reading LEAN HAPPY HEALTHY YOU to extend self-discovery. You can use the CAMP OUT WITH THE LEAN HAPPY HEALTHY YOU JOURNAL that accompanies this book.

A quick aside for what's next:
The RiTual *is also called* **The RiT***.*

2. Practice the habits right away. The only way to let *The RiT* improve your health and reduce body fat is by practicing the 8 habits immediately and consistently.

This is a reference book *and* a book of action steps. This book requires movement.

Get up right now. Wave your arms in the air. Shake your hips to the four corners of the universe. Pretend you hear music. Shake it, stir it, wiggle up and down. Okay, have a seat. Just checking to see if you're ready to take the cue to move.

Implement each of the habits immediately after you read them. Reading doesn't deliver understanding. Practice does.

I estimate you'll be able to finish this book in a couple weeks. Within four weeks you'll look, feel, and rest better. Within twelve weeks other folks will notice you've lost body-fat. Within a year you'll notice you've kept the fat lost, and you'll feel like a revived version of yourself.

3. Practice *The RiT* by **sharing it with someone else.**
Keep in mind, there's no way you'll become an authority for a process or system you haven't thoroughly

embodied. So before you teach someone what you've learned in this book, take notes and practice the 8 habits of *The RiT* for yourself.

Witness your own transformation and you'll be naturally inclined to go out and ambassador the habits. When folks ask how you got so lean and energetic, you'll be able to share these tools along with your personal story.

Folks are gonna notice that you avoid the temptations in your environment that used to have you by the chin. Tell them you have a *RiTual* of healthy habits that you live every day. Or better, buy someone their own copy of LEAN HAPPY HEALTHY YOU and practice the 8 healthy habits with them.

You're on our way, but first let me tell you why I wanna help you.

• • •

In every block of marble I see a statue as plain as though it
stood before me, shaped and perfect in attitude and action.
I have only to hew away the rough walls that imprison the
lovely apparition to reveal it to the other eyes as mine see it.

the intuitive artist, Michelangelo

PART ONE

IDENTITY

I HATE EXERCISE

I dissolved my *can't*, embodied *CAN*, and changed
my future.

I had to be the least likely woman to become a fitness
professional. I didn't wear sneakers till my twenties
because I didn't consider them cute shoes. During my
youth, I could polish off man-sized servings of anything.
Plus, I frickn loathed exercise.

In high school I was a perky pom-pom girl and a
dramatic singer. Short bursts of dancing was the closest I
got to exercising. Pretending I was one of Prince's
pupils, with my faux fur vest and my hair swept to one
side to expose two-inch feather earrings, I clearly
preferred *dressing up* to *sweating out*. I grew up in Iowa.
I was a bored there, I mean I was *creative* there.
Anyway, to think my style could be cramped by sweaty
hair and extreme exertion made exercising a situation I
avoided like a pothole.

Gym class was mandatory. I was forced to fake
basketball. I still harbor an intense anger for the schmuck
who created dodgeball. Jogging around that red, hellish
track bordered on corporal punishment.

We had to pass swimming to graduate. I swam every
day of summer when I was younger though in a much
smaller body. I knew how to swim just fine. What were
high school level swim lessons gonna teach me? I was
especially sensitive because it was a co-ed class. I had
to wear my swimsuit without a covering in front of the
boys.

My hate for gym class grew horns.

I'd escape Phys Ed through out-of-body projections. I'd
mind-plop into my fantasies for 45 minutes. When that
didn't work, I'd find a partner who felt just as
embarrassed as I, and we'd cling to each other in
conversation about anything other than what was going
on in P.E.

When we had to do straight leg lifts for warm-ups,
Mr. Tim didn't bother to explain *how* to do them.
I couldn't lift my legs off the ground. I'd lie on the mat,
legs flopping, pretending I was invisible or in my fantasy
with Donna Summer or Barbra Streisand.

Twice a year my school held fit tests—a bane of my
contempt for gym. I'd roll my eyes and click my

sneakers three times—*ANYWHERE BUT HERE, ANYWHERE BUT HERE, ANYWHERE BUT HERE.*

The worst exercise was the pull-up-and-hold required for the girls. I'd pull, almost snapping my arm out of socket to try to get off the chair that gave us a boost. My best friend tucked her chin over that bar, turned purple and shook for two minutes. The class applauded her. I felt like a big loser. How did she hold her weight at the bar, but I hung at the bottom? We wore each other's clothes, for doggone sake. Shouldn't I be as strong?

The sit-ups were barf-worthy. The amped athletic kids turned green and hammered endless sit-ups. Their eyes spun for the thrill of running, pulling, and crunching hysterics. I was amped for performance—singing, dancing, and being glamorous. I found no delight in panting, grimacing, or wiping eye liner sweat down my cheek. I wasn't made to be fit, and I hated being judged with a grade C in gym for being myself.

I was an eater. Of everything. Really, everything, except peas and liver. That was my thing. If you put anything in front of me that didn't have peas or liver in it, it'd be gone in a blink. My family branded this problem *funny.*

My eating habit was further intensified by their constant teasing.

The gorging started in middle school. I'd wait till I was alone in the kitchen with the leftovers. Washing the dishes gave me private time to complete the gorge.

I was an expert at devouring bread. Biscuits didn't stand a chance in my kitchen. I delighted in raw foods, too. Not raw carrots or celery... raw cookie dough, cake batter, and brownie batter. I knew nothing of salmonella. I've eaten so many raw eggs, I'm probably immune to it.

Desperate to beat the fat from consuming my body during senior year, I situated a pill-and-soda habit. My best friend and I would fill 64-ounce Big Gulps with diet Pepsi and chug 'em with yellow pills for breakfast and lunch. After school, we'd attack a Dairy Queen dessert, barf (or at least try) then sing at her house.

Year upon year the circumference of my legs ballooned while my belly folds rolled like the high seas. By college I was eating as much as a boy on an Olympic wrestling team. I needed to do something. I needed to arrest what life, food, and gravity were doing to my body and my taste buds.

Cellulite formed soft shelves on my hips. I attempted to jog hoping it'd banish the 20 pounds I'd gained by my second year of college. I heard running worked the fastest. I put aside my disdain for sweaty hair and hit the pavement. At twenty minutes-a-run, it worked. My saddle hips smoothed down, so I stopped running and crossed my fingers. I gained the weight back in a month.

This is the body I've been given. I'm a Big Girl and I love food. Nothing will change that.

This was the one thing I knew for sure, the one thing I loathed about myself.

By age 23, I wished for a fairy godmother to transform me. On a clear day in Chicago when Spring had finally let Summer have her way, I reluctantly slipped into large white tennis shorts and a tank. My boyfriend was outside on the front stoop of our greystone chatting-up a buddy. I went down to join them. They paused when I came into view. Both grew stiffly silent. Two sets of eyes hit my fat legs like heat, and I swoll with an embarrassment I'll never forget.

I'd stopped paying attention to my weight. I hadn't looked into a full-length mirror in years. I'd given up on the weight-loss shenanigans. I'd been focusing on graduating, moving to a new city, leaving loads of friends, and figuring out how to grow up and make money. The whole time I'd kept eating and eating and eating.

The silent judgment pierced an IV into my chest. I could hear their criticisms pump like an infusion—*Does she know she looks like that? How did she get so big? Damn, she's out of shape. She's got a lot of nerve to leave the house like that. Why doesn't she just wear a skirt?*

I wanted to disappear, run upstairs and get a skirt, cry. I heard a whimper. It was me sighing the truth: *I am gonna get bigger, fatter, and more out of control and I have no idea how to stop it or make the fat to go away.*

Time froze that day. Nothing changed either. I ran upstairs and put on a skirt.

I met Elliot when I got hired to sing in Osaka, Japan a year later. Our cast of eight splashed around the fabulous hotel pool after rehearsal.

Elliot whispered—*You have a nice shape, Michelle.* He saw my body after I finally peeled the sarong from my waist. We'd been dancing in rehearsals every day for two weeks since we arrived in Japan. My body looked better than the hot mess it was before the gig started.

Elliot's words felt like a compliment—sort of. I knew he meant *I have a nice shape for a BIG GIRL.*

My 23-year-old heart laughed and splashed out a *thank you*, though every cell inside echoed whimpers of the pain that conversations about weight always made me feel. *Nice shape? Sure. I would never look like the other two girls in our group.*

The other two ladies were gymnasts with beautiful muscles like professional dancers. The difference was undeniable when our outfits for the show were selected by the staff. The dancer ladies were given tiny black shorts and sneakers, while I wore 3/4 length shorts, over thick lace tights.

During a private lunch with Elliot, he confronted my weight. No one had talked about my weight without a punchline. Elliot didn't chuckle.

Michelle, you are young and attractive. You're a soprano, so you're gonna be cast to play the ingenues. If you keep gaining weight you'll be playing mamas in a year, and that's only if you can sing the part. You have to decide what you want for yourself. If you don't want to lose weight for vanity, you'd better try to do it for your career.

Everyone can lose weight, Michelle. The reason they don't is because they can't see themselves differently. Michelle, I see you shapely and tight. You have beautiful legs and a nice torso. Lose that extra fat and it will change everything for you—especially the way you feel about yourself.

I lost my appetite. A good feeling came into my body. Elliot revealed the yellow bricks. He dropped a rainbow into view.

I shook myself back to Kansas. I was born with big bones. Other family members had weight issues like mine. Both my parents had high blood pressure. *I'm supposed to be this way,* I convinced myself.

I could never control my appetite, anyway. The smell of food was a bell that made me salivate. I hated the absurdity of my over-eating, like I was a caged animal set free over a trough where I'd slurp and inhale grub, trying not to let my hair fall into the food. I wondered how it felt to be full. I had no idea. The food needed to be gone before I'd stop eating. Gone.

I've tried exercise, Elliot. It doesn't work for me... My typical excuse lunged from my lips. Elliot had his palm up, ready.

He told me his weight-loss story and how it pushed him to become an aerobic teacher. His weight-loss opened other opportunities for him. He was cast in THE FIRM workout videos from the 80s and 90s because of his commitment. A gang of aerobic students awaited his return from our 8-week gig in Japan. Elliot told me I could do the same thing. I could change my body starting now, and that if I did, it would open my life beyond my imagination.

Thank you sir Elliot, wherever you are, for your rawness and rightness and blatant honesty. I needed you to challenge my limiting beliefs. You made me confront the fears I'd rolled into excuses. I had been willing to accept a definition of myself that made me feel embarrassed, ashamed, and mis-represented. Elliott was the first person who ever said I was good enough to have a healthy, fit body. I needed to know I was good enough. I needed to hear I was good enough to believe I could feel confident in my body.

When I returned from Japan, I went to see Anna.

The Spanish, Russian, and English-speaking, thick-bodied, thick-accented, forcefully loud, Polish aerobic instructor, my aerobic instructor. Anna.

You're not gonna lose that weight like that, Michelle. Get off that treadmill and into my class!

That was the gist of our first interaction.

Anna had already lost 100 pounds, and with just 30 pounds more to lose, she was the most determined instructor in the gym. Back then most aerobic instructors were skinny girls. This was during the early 90s.
I had a hard time believing those naturally skinny aerobic instructors could understand my plight—that I ate without a gauge and that I found it impossible to catch my breath after 10 minutes of exercise. I wanted to be instructed by a fellow BIG GIRL who knew my struggles.

I let Anna yell at me four days a week... "Go, go... 4, 3, 2, 1!"

The first month sucked. I attended her classes, arriving late each time, and stopping after 10-15 minutes. They were all-out kick-butt minutes, though. I'd give my 15-minute all-out effort till I couldn't breathe, then retreat to the treadmill. Three months later, I stood front and center with Anna for the whole hour.

Twenty pounds slimmer, I bumped into a dude in Woolworth's who almost dropped his purchase when he saw me.
Anna's classes did this to me, I told him.

I shifted. On the inside. I believed it was possible to change, then I shifted. I set a goal to lose 20 pounds. I locked into a consistent workout schedule, jamming with Anna four days a week, adding easier classes two days a week. The six days of exercise worked magic on my appetite. I didn't have to rein in my trough-style urges. Because of my commitment to aerobics with Anna, I craved healthier food and less of it.

I imagined my body changed before it happened. After class, when the aerobic studio was cleared out, I'd stand before the wall of mirrors and scan my body. I'd rotate and sculpt my body mentally. I'd imagine firm legs, slim arms, and a flat stomach. The image wasn't real in the mirror, it was real in my mind. I saw the future I intended.

Months passed. A year passed. I changed. Everyone noticed.

I know how it feels to hate exercise. I know how it feels to resist it, to feel overwhelmed by it.

When I focused solely on what I hated, the sweat and exertion, it only expanded those feelings. It put me on a hamster wheel of wanting a change while despising and loathing that I wouldn't commit to change.

Elliot suggested I take a big-vision approach and imagine how my career and confidence would improve. **Elliot told me he believed in me.** He took my life seriously, so I took my vision seriously. It worked.

I cherish what my body has been able to do. I'm amazed by the power of my mind. I'm sure my healthy habits are saving my life and I want to share these habits with you. Let's focus on what you need to know so you can go for what you intend.

• • •

My mission in life is not merely to survive, but to thrive; and to
do so with some passion, some compassion, some humor,
and some style.

the Wise Mother of the soulful word, Maya Angelou

I HAVE NO IDEA HOW THE WEIGHT FELL OFF

If you've lost weight on a program in the past but managed to put more weight on within the year, **you didn't learn how to lose weight effectively.** If you spend four hours in the gym, seven days a week, **you haven't figured out how to lose weight properly** (unless you're a professional athlete). If you've packed your freezer with frozen TV dinners and packed your pantry with gluten-free cookies, crackers, and pasta, **you might not know how to stay healthy and lose weight.** If you signed a contract to take an 18-day 100% juice cleanse to lose 25 pounds for your class reunion only to re-gain 32 pounds two months later, **you didn't lose weight effectively.**

Skipping meals to speed your weight-loss and working out every day while feasting on microwavable burritos and diet soda is not going to spark good health or improve weight-loss confidence. If you've lost weight before but can't explain *how* you did it, you don't understand how to lose weight and keep it off.

Of the many philosophies out there, the one you're probably familiar with is MOVE MORE, EAT LESS. Eat less of what? Is walking my dog enough movement? It's a start, but this bit of logic is only a teeny part of the solution.

Uh-oh, Stacy.

Stacy didn't learn how to lose weight and keep it off.

Stacy MOVED MORE and ATE a lot LESS. It made her skinny-fat. Her intense workouts required better nutrition, including fiber-rich carbs for energy, essential fats for her joints, and protein to build lean muscle. Instead, she under-ate and lost weight so fast, it left her saggy, barely strong, and lacking energy. The improper intake of nutrition and water along with an inadequate amount sleep tanked her immune system.

Stacy needed to eat more, nourish more, drink more water, lift weights more, and rest more.

"I know exactly what to do to lose this weight, Michelle. I just don't do it."

I hear this often. Maybe, it's true. Maybe not so much. There are three reasons people say things like this and then later admit they can't seem to follow-through and lose weight.

1. They do not know what to do at all.
2. They might know what to do, but can't imagine themselves fit or lean.
3. They believe the weight is helping them manage an issue or role in their life.

Do you identify with any of these?

• • •

In any given moment we have two options: to step forward
into growth or step back into safety.

Abraham Maslow
legendary teacher of personal growth

Your feelings can either be the biggest deterrent to achieving your weight-loss goal or choosing your desired feelings can march you right over the finish-line. Point your mind and your desired feeling at your goal.

Jump into the future.

Focus on the way you want to feel when you've reached your goal. Think less about whether you will, can, or can't lose weight. Don't even think about how you'll be able to maintain the fat-loss after you lose it. **Simply consider the desired feeling you want to experience when it happens.**

How do you want to feel when you lose the excess weight?

Can you anchor yourself to this desired feeling even when other feelings bully for your attention?

Tony Robbins says the drive behind most choices is an inherent desire to feel pleasure and avoid pain. Your perception of pleasure and pain determines your level of commitment.

If you think having moderately sore muscles for three days is **too** painful, you'll avoid a strength training program that promises stronger bones and an efficient metabolism. If you think missing an episode of *Dancing with the Stars* is unbearable, you won't go to the evening Zumba class to dance, laugh, and relieve stress. If you believe it's inconvenient to stock-up on veggies, pickles, and grass-fed beef from the farmer's market on Saturday, you'll order a Domino's pizza on your next stressed-out weekend.

If you believe it **painful** to shift your habits and up-level the way you see yourself, you won't stand a chance when you face big obstacles along your fat-loss path. Once again...

How do you want to feel when you lose the excess weight?
How will feeling this way change your life?

Write your thoughts.

When I carried excess weight, I also harbored a low
opinion about my worth. I was a singer for most of my
youth. I experienced vocal problems in my early twenties,
right before graduating from college. I didn't lose my
singing voice completely, but my vocal power was
significantly reduced. I kept singing even though I didn't
sound as good as before, in my opinion. No one knew
I'd sounded better years earlier except those who'd
heard me sing before my voice changed. My potency as
a person was tied to my vocal confidence. Through
journaling I discovered I binged as a form of grieving.
Through journaling I realized that both singing and over-
eating masked my hurt around daddy issues, boyfriend
issues, and not-enoughness issues. The body-fat
insulated me though I never felt FULL. Journaling helped
me realize that the more I ate, the more I felt sad, angry,
and worthless. My foot was nailed to a floor of HUNGER.
I was destined to run in circles until I addressed the
reasons *why* I ate so much.

After I dropped 20 pounds with Anna, I started
performing regularly again. The singing gifted me
opportunities to live my dreams. I got cast in the second

national tour of the Broadway musical, Once On This
Island. I played a sixteen year-old girl in love, cast partly
because I looked 10 years younger after losing weight.
(Elliot was right) Singing availed other dreams to come
true. I created a drama program and a Yoga program for
children through The City University of New York. I
developed the Theatre department at a high school in
the South Bronx. The courage I used to focus on losing
the weight gave me the discipline and stamina for other
visions. The discipline of losing excess weight could
cause other areas of your life to flourish.

The journaling questions throughout this book help you
understand if excess weight protects you, justifies a
particular role you've unconsciously chosen, or resigns
you to the limiting beliefs you hold about yourself.
If you're ready to confront your beliefs and construct a
new definition of yourself, you'll do great in this program.

*How do you expect to feel when you are living a healthy,
fit, courageous life?*

Whatever you wrote—this is the dominant feeling you
must focus on when the other feelings battle to force you
from your dream.

• • •

Knowing how you actually want to feel is the most potent form
of clarity that you can have.
Generating those feelings is the most powerfully creative thing
you can do with your life.

When you get clear on how you want to feel,
the pursuit itself will become more satisfying.

Danielle LaPorte,
succulent poet and teacher,
the author of The Desire Map and The Firestarter Sessions

We're in the beginning

of an over-fat epidemic in America, but we *can* turn it into a happier, healthier "middle".

The following data massively turns my stomach.
As of 2014, 30% of women were overweight. In 2018, 35% of the U.S. population was overweight. Okay, that's a lot of folks. And here's the thing: I know *overweight* can be misrepresented when total body composition isn't considered. Your total body composition includes the weight of your fat + lean muscle tissue + your organs + the thickness of your bones. Yes, you can be a few pounds heavier because of thicker, denser bones, and muscle. You can calculate your body fat percentage by using skin-fold calipers. Most gyms have someone on staff who can take these measurements for you.
I recommend using a tape measure and logging the circumference of certain body sites. I'll show you how to do this in PART FOUR along with other ways to track your progress. I do not recommend using a scale to weigh yourself often at all.

Here's why. Most statistics define a woman up to 5' 9" weighing between 169 – 202 pounds as overweight. Any woman (5'9" and shorter) over 203 lbs is

considered medically obese. More than 30 pounds
overweight is considered obese.

Okay ladies, champion tennis player Serena Williams is
5' 9" and weighs between 170-200 pounds. Lindsey
Vonn, the champion skier, is 5' 10" and weighs 160 lbs.
These ladies barely clear the label *overweight*. They have
elite cardiovascular stamina and muscular strength. When
I competed in three bodybuilding shows, I weighed
between 139-141 pounds at 5' 4 ½". According to my
doctor's chart, my competition weight should have been
my everyday weight. At 141 pounds my body was
ripped. My face was sunken. My eyes appeared oversized. Now I'm at my desirable weight range of 149-154
lbs, which is considered 5 lbs overweight for my height.
I wear a size small to medium dress, a size 6 pant, and I
don't have any medical prescriptions to fill. I'm lean with
sculpted muscle. I rarely catch a cold and take an aspirin
once or twice a year. I only mention this because I don't
want you to assume your "actual weight" is a point of
concern. Be clear that excess body fat that accumulates
around the abdominal area is a primary health concern.
Being either over-fat or obese around the middle is the
issue we must take much more seriously than scale
weight.

A waist measurement greater than 35 inches may be considered over fat and at medium risk for heart disease and Type II Diabetes. Joint problems due to obesity is another concern.

Type I diabetes is an autoimmune disease typified by an unresponsive pancreas. It accounts for 5-10% of diabetes cases and it's usually diagnosed in juvenile years. The proper role of the pancreas is to produce insulin to handle the sugars from your food. Insulin pushes the sugars, or glucose, into your cells. The pancreas does not respond at all in those who have Type I Diabetes. Instead, the individual must inject insulin after every meal.

My dad had Type I Diabetes. When an individual with Diabetes Type I does not regulate the glucose into the cells, they could face circulatory problems, impaired vision, and the risk of heart disease and stroke.

If you have Type I Diabetes, you **must** eat healthy, low-sugar meals at regular intervals every day of your life. And you must inject insulin when eating to stay alive. You cannot cure Type I Diabetes.

Type II Diabetes, however, is an acquired disease. The precursor is an issue of **insulin resistance** caused by behaviors you *can* control including excessive belly-fat, high sugar meals, inactivity, sleep disorders, excessive diseases and medications, imbalances of hormones, and cigarette smoking. You can prevent Type II Diabetes by amending the lifestyle habits that cause it. You'll amend those habits by practicing *The RiT.*

Type II Diabetes used to be a disease attributed to adults. Disturbingly, the cases in children have increased from 5% in 1994 to 20% most recently.

Statistics on their own can feel impersonal. But these are personal to me. Just writing this makes me want do 20 jumping jacks and eat a bouquet of carrots.

An epidemic. This is really happening folks. If my mind and body hadn't been turned around by Elliot, I'd be lumped into these stats. *How do you feel about them?*

DECIDE

Decide **you** are not going to flirt with these health risks. Decide you do not want to be a part of this bad news tribe! Decide you are done deferring your goal. You're

done hoping, wishing, dreaming, and one-daying your
health and body vision.

Commit.

Practice the healthy habits for your mind, heart, and body
starting now. Make the decision that you won't let
discomfort or temporary pain upstage your dedication to
your Self. This will be a life-saving decision.

PART TWO

FOCUS

• • •

Great accomplishment does not come by being random.

Michelle Bernard

THE CHARLIE BROWN SOLUTION

Have you seen Charlie Brown's closet? Every hanger holds a yellow shirt with a black zig zag near the hem. There's nothing else hanging in there. Charlie Brown, the existential PEANUT with GOOD GRIEF, has managed to conquer one of his woes. He doesn't have to figure out what he's gonna wear each day.

President Obama owned suits in two colors: blue and gray. Steve Jobs wore black turtlenecks and jeans every day. Mark Zuckerberg probably owns drawers of gray hoodies because that's what he's seen wearing most of the time. Obama, the late Jobs, and Zuckerberg shared three commonalities: the drive to succeed, a desire to impact other's lives, and the wherewithal to automate a daily habit that otherwise would have sucked extra mental energy.

Making new decisions all day
can be exhausting.

DECISION FATIGUE

or I'll take one in every color—can I do that?

Matilda Kahl has to make important decisions at her New York ad agency. Decision-making started in her bountiful closet. What will she wear to work? *Maybe the blue ones...? Or the green pair... Where's the other...? Did I dry-clean those plaid slacks? Shucks. These blacks don't match.*

After a typical morning of wrestling to pick an outfit, Kahl arrived at work late and frustrated. That was the last day she let her energy dehydrate in her closet.

Kahl deferred to **The Charlie Brown Solution**. She purchased fifteen identical white blouses and five pairs of black slacks. She wears this combo to work. Every day. She's been asked if wearing the same outfit daily is boring. She compared dressing for work to scheduling automatic bill-pay in an article for Harper's Bazaar.

"You know, with confidence, your bills are paid on time."

By automating a deliriously taxing daily decision, Kahl saves time and mental energy.

Kahl, President Obama, Zuckerberg, and the late Jobs utilized **The Charlie Brown Solution**: AUTOMATE THE DECISIONS THAT TAX YOUR ENERGY AND WILLPOWER.

You will also automate the 8 HEALTHY HABITS, *The RiTual.* It'll reduce your worry and confusion about what to eat, do, and believe every day. When these healthy habits become your automatic behaviors, you'll use less mental energy to implement them. They'll give your healthy life a sense of predictability and ease.

Your current body and state of health are a result of the habits that have given your life predictability. Maybe you don't consciously know what those habits are. One of my clients confessed to visiting Dunkin Donuts before work every morning. What did she order? A medium coffee with three sugars, cream, and oh yeah, a chocolate glazed donut—every morning.

"I guess I'm a creature of habit," she giggled.

I had a client who'd wait in a deli line out the door, because she *had* to have her small coffee, sweet and lite, and a freshly-made bagel with veggie cream cheese before work. If the line moved slowly, oh the anger and frustration. She'd rather risk being late for work than skip her bagel. Skipping out on your daily routine could ruin your mood.

Think about the habitual behaviors that bring a sense of certainty to your day. *How would you feel if these habits got interrupted?* Probably lost. Maybe upset. Slightly uncomfortable.

Do you have a nightly routine that helps you prepare for work or school the next day?

Perhaps this routine ensures fewer hiccups in the morning. Think of things you do the same way every morning.

Do you travel the same route to work or school?

Perhaps you trust the route to get you there on-time or it keeps you from getting lost.

Do you have a Saturday or Sunday routine?

Perhaps you pick-up your clothes from the dry cleaners, wash the car, visit family members, worship in church, or exercise during weekend mornings. You hold your

weekend routines sacred. Running weekend errands
helps the weekdays flow efficiently.

**Take a moment and consider the answers to the
questions above. Jot your responses in your journal.**

ROUTINES REQUIRE LESS ENERGY

Charles Duhigg, author of The Power of Habits, reported
that 40-45% of the decisions we make each day are
habitual because they require less energy. For example,
Duhigg observed a rat's movement through a maze to
get to a piece of chocolate placed in the center. The rat
wandered the maze sniffing, scratching, and hunting for
the chocolate. It took the rat thirteen minutes to find it.
The researcher was able to track the rat's mental activity
during the hunt. The graph lit up when the rat scratched
at the walls. The needle scribbled wildly when the rat
found the chocolate.

The experiment was tracked repeatedly and the rat found
the chocolate faster each time. With each attempt, the
graph registered less mental activity from the rat. The rat
was using less brain power to figure out how to get the

chocolate because its brain had routinized or
programmed the exercise. The happy rat got to his
reward with greater ease when the exercise had become
a habit.

Excellence is an art won by training and habituation: we do not
act right because we have virtue or excellence, but we rather
have these because we have acted rightly...

We are what we repeatedly do.
Excellence, then, is not an act,
but a habit.

Aristotle

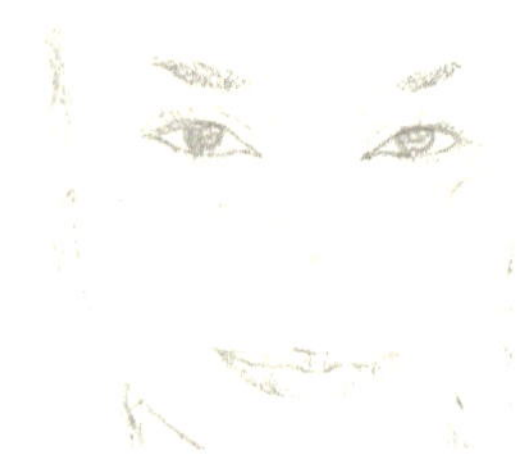

h.a.b.i.t.

harness your creative mind

abandon your barriers

bring a desired vision and feeling into your body

initiate a series of behaviors that align with your

vision

IN ORDER TO EXPERIENCE A

transformation that is sustainable.

Most folks who want to lose fat will focus on healthy habits for their body. You are more than a body. If you have found it difficult to lose fat or keep the fat lost, it's likely you haven't integrated healthy **h.a.b.i.t.s** for both your mind and heart.

h.a.b.i.t.

harness your
creative mind.

You have a powerful mind. **Your thoughts can either strengthen your body or weaken it.**

I was selected out of a live audience to demonstrate the correlation between my thoughts and my body through a muscle testing experiment. Perhaps the speaker chose me because my tank top showed I had strong-looking arms.

I extended my right arm out at shoulder height. The presenter asked me an easy question. I answered MICHELLE as she pushed down on my forearm and wrist. No movement. I felt the resistance, but I was able to withstand the weight of her pressure.

After, she told me to answer with a fake name.

I answered NANCY. She pushed. My strong arm
withered and fell, almost all the way to my side. The
audience choked. Me too. I mean, what was that? Her
effort of push didn't match the amount of weight I could
lift in the gym.
My arm was weak when I lied.

With the next few questions, she had me switch arms so
fatigue wouldn't be a factor. **I AM GRATEFUL TO BE
ALIVE.** Strong arm. No movement. **LIFE IS HARD.** Arm
lost control and moved down to my side again.
I said the word: **PROCRASTINATION.** Weak arm.
Procrastinating is a problem for me sometimes. The word
has a weakening energy.

Muscle testing showed how negative intentions and false
statements weakened my body. Truthful statements and
positive intentions strengthened my body. This is
probably true for you.

Everyone has inner conversations. What do you tell
yourself about your health, your shape, and your physical
abilities?
How do you think your inner conversation is affecting
your body and your weight?

I hate my legs, My body sucks, I get fat if I look at lasagna.
Come on girl—just one more lap. Nothing can stop me!
Wow, I look good this week. That was the best set of push ups I've ever done.

How do you speak to yourself?

POINT OF FOCUS

Life flows between high points and low points, challenges and victories. Sometimes you'll coast. Other times you'll freeze. You respond to these fluctuations based on how you perceive them. Other people respond from their perspective. **Your overall belief about yourself and life informs where you choose to place your focus.**

I've represented the three areas of the creative mind based on its characteristic. The subconscious mind is the PROGRAM. The conscious mind is the PRINCIPLE mind, and superconsciousness is POSSIBILITY.

Take a breath, then exhale. Do it again, but this time inhale slower, and exhale even slower. Do it three more times with relaxed eyes.
Now tune in to the sounds around you.

Listen. What do you hear?

What else do you hear?

Close your eyes and listen for another minute.

Open your eyes and keep listening to the sounds for one more minute.

Take another slow breath in, then exhale slowly.

Your PRINCIPLE mind just did that exercise. You **paid attention** to the directives using your conscious mind. You became aware using your senses and thoughts. Your PRINCIPLE mind is the creative mind that pays attention. It also scrutinizes and make inferences based on the data stored in your PROGRAM, your subconscious mind.

Your PRINCIPLE mind may have inferred that I'd ask you to take the last breath slowly, because I gave you that cue earlier. You PROGRAMMED that cue or remembered it (from a past experience).

YOU'VE PROGRAMMED A SET OF BELIEFS ABOUT YOUR BODY

You have more than **50,000** thoughts every day. Most of them are recycled thoughts from yesterday and the day before. When you replay a particular thought often, it inspires a feeling that also gets replayed. Your feelings live in your body, so thoughts affect the body through feelings.

When a repeated thought inspires a corresponding feeling often enough, it imprints a belief into your mind.

Let's say you start a workout program **thinking**: *I am so tired, I can hardly breathe. I really hate working out. I wish I could get liposuction for my belly instead of sweating like this.*

Those thoughts inspire these corresponding **feelings**: *It's been three weeks of exercise and I feel* **hopeless** *because I'm still out of breath. I'm* **embarrassed** *because my body hasn't improved yet. I'm sore after the workouts and haven't lost any of this belly–fat. I'm* **angry.** *My arms hurt for nothing.*

Your PROGRAM or the subconscious mind registers this **belief**: *Working out doesn't do anything for me. It makes me sore and it doesn't change the way I look. It's a waste of time.*

Your beliefs influence your decisions which determine how committed you'll be during your healthy lifestyle program.

If you make a decision to hire a personal trainer, but you believe it's too hard for you to lose weight, **you will not lose weight.** You unconsciously want to make your beliefs true. By "you", I mean—**your body and mind** want your beliefs to be true. Your body and mind will align with the intentions of your beliefs in order to validate them, especially when your belief is repeated regularly and often in your mind.

Let's look closer into your PROGRAM of thoughts, the place where your beliefs get incubated.

THE PROGRAM

Ninety-five percent of your daily behavior is influenced by the thoughts and beliefs in your PROGRAM. Your subconscious mind, the PROGRAM, is filled to the brim with memories and other input from your past experiences. Music, movies, and television, and other sensory information is saved in your PROGRAM.

Your PROGRAM is not interested in whether any of your stored data is healthy or dangerous for you. It stores and informs you based on what you've chosen to focus on most, both mentally and emotionally.

Once your PROGRAM establishes beliefs, you lean on them as guidelines. You may not be aware you're doing it either. If you've had a difficult time losing weight, you probably have a belief that supports that weight-loss is difficult.

You can change a belief. Beliefs are not absolute facts. They are your facts based on perceptions you've thought repeatedly, focused on, and felt most often. When you change sabotaging thoughts and feelings, you change your beliefs. That's when you can change your outcomes.

Here are a few mental PROGRAMS that support an elevated state of health.

1. I'm honestly a happy person. I was made that way.
2. There are only two things I'm afraid of: Not putting forth effort to make my goals work and living with regret because I was afraid to go for my dreams.

3. I cannot solve a problem if I let my mind ruminate
    over the problem. I'm the type who focuses on
    the solution.
4. I keep picturing myself on the beach in that
    yellow bikini with a big smile across my face.
5. I go to the gym to workout even when I don't
    want to because I ALWAYS feel better afterward.

If you hold your arm out to muscle test these beliefs,
you'll be a powerhouse.

Here are a few PROGRAMS (habits of thought) that can
sabotage your health goals. Your arm would wither to
your side if you spoke these beliefs.

1. Based on my genetics, I'll probably be obese well
    past my 30s.
2. I experience too many set-backs to be able to .
    thrive on a weight-loss program.
3. It's gonna be impossible to eat healthy when I
    take my business trips because of the client
    dinners.
4. I hope my boyfriend doesn't feel uncomfortable
    because I'm watching what I eat. It's going to
    cause me more aggravation than it's worth to eat
    healthy when I'm around him.

5. I'm not perfect.

Even *I'm not perfect* is a sabotaging belief. Say those words: *I'm not perfect.* How do they make you feel? *I'm not perfect* weakens your body. It resonates as *I'm not whole, I'm not ready,* and *I'm not full.* Those words also presuppose that someone actually *is* perfect and compared to *that perfect person*, you are far less capable. Therefore, your mind believes that *if you are far less capable*, you have permission to demonstrate insufficiency. Perfection is not applicable to humans, anyway. POSSIBILITY is. I'll discuss POSSIBILITY as you read on.

How can you up-level your PROGRAM and change your beliefs to support your goals?

1. You could try hypnosis. Hypnosis is a mental intervention that interrupts and extracts sabotaging beliefs, then rewrites new thoughts into your PROGRAM.
2. Tapping or E.F.T., the Emotional Freedom Technique. This is a healing technique whereby you tap on meridian sites while speaking through your negative beliefs and negative emotions. You

keep speaking and tapping until you can speak beliefs that support you.

3. The other way to change your PROGRAM is by engaging in routine behaviors and inner conversations reinforced by positive emotions and rewards (like the rat experienced). That's what we're gonna do.

Tracy thought it nearly impossible to lose weight. If she looked at food she'd get fat. She hated the gym but was willing to give it another try this year.

Tracy set a resolution to lose 25 pounds. She started taking Zumba classes on January 5th with a friend from work. They'd chat on Sunday night. Her friend would remind Tracy to pack workout clothes for Monday.

For the first 3 weeks, they made it to 4 classes every week. Even though Tracy felt a little sore because she hadn't worked out in years, she never missed a Zumba class. Her jeans got looser. She could pull her belt one notch tighter. Tracy's friend kept her consistent.

On the 4th week, Tracy's friend forgot her clothes. Tracy decided she'd take an evening walk instead of going to Zumba alone. After dinner Tracy's boyfriend called. She hung up at 10 pm. Tracy skipped the walk, stuck a bag

of popcorn in the microwave, and watched reruns of
Scandal till bedtime.
By the end of the week, Tracy had taken Zumba class
once. The following week, she skipped Zumba because
her friend's work schedule changed.

Even though Tracy got favorable results from exercising,
it didn't motivate her to commit to a consistent schedule.
When her circumstances changed, Tracy re-aligned with
her old PROGRAM of thoughts.
I don't like the gym. I hate working out alone. It's
impossible to lose weight. I get fat when I look at food.

Her subconscious PROGRAM took over, as it usually
does.

1. Tracy needed to **imagine** how her life would improve
   from being fit and healthy.
2. She needed a **plan of daily habits** to combat her
   mental obstacles.
3. She needed to set **meaningful goals** and define the
   way she ultimately desired to feel once her vision
   became reality.
4. Tracy needed to **journal** about her emotional obstacles
   and write her visions every day.

Think about your past efforts, present fears, and personal challenges associated with losing fat, starting an exercise program, and eating healthy.

Whatever poses great difficulty, an obstacle, or aversion for you is connected to a belief you have PROGRAMMED in your subconscious mind.

It doesn't matter how or when you PROGRAMMED. It only matters that you become aware it exists.
You can change it.

CHOOSE YOUR PRINCIPLES

You are conscious 5-10% of the time every day. Eek! That's not much. Most of your mental behavior is on autopilot. Most of your daily behaviors are habituated by your PROGRAM.

Have you ever driven your car to work all the while reliving your dinner date? *Matthew picked the most elegant restaurant on the rooftop of the hotel overlooking the Hudson River. The sky was purple and orange as the sun slipped into the water. The fennel salad with a*

*splash of citrus vinaigrette was divine. He was so
adorable in that blue suit and pink tie.* Wait. Who's
driving your car right now? Your PRINCIPLE mind is
paying attention to Saturday night, but somehow you just
made it to work in one piece. Who was driving your car
while you were forming beliefs about how much your
guy loves you? Your PROGRAM.

You've been driving for 20 years. You've driven the
same route every day for 10 years. You can drive on
autopilot. You don't have to dedicate 100% of your
mental attention to driving unless you visit a new town or
if you're new to driving a stick (the cramp in your foot
will go away eventually).

Every time your PRINCIPLE mind gets called to analyze,
reason, or recall; your PROGRAM clicks into autopilot.
Your PROGRAM clicks into autopilot 90–95% of the time.

Think of all the things you did today on autopilot. Were
you totally present as you brushed your teeth? When
you showered? As you put on your shoes? Think of the
times when you were PAYING ATTENTION today.
Crickets. It takes longer to think of the these times. You
must consciously pay attention when you study for a test.
To learn a new dance step—you must be fully

conscious. To learn a new language, you must pay full
attention.

You enact most of your day from your PROGRAM.
This explains why you unconsciously repeat old habits
like noshing on the Ritz crackers after dinner and
grabbing two doughnuts when you stop for your morning
coffee. Your PROGRAM reminds you to do what you
"always do".

To change your body you will PAY ATTENTION to new
ways of being—new habits. After much repetition, the
new habits, the habit of *The RiT,* will become
PROGRAMMED. When this happens your life and body
will change.

• • •

We see the world, not as it is, but as we are—,

or,

as we are conditioned to see it.

Stephen Covey, author of the renowned productivity book,

The 7 Habits of Highly Effective People

WHAT'S POSSIBLE?

POSSIBILITY mind is an underutilized gift. The superconscious mind, POSSIBILITY, is where most children play.

What if any outcome you intended were possible?

How would you choose to experience a healthy love relationship? As an exercise, imagine you could have the kind of love you truly wanted. *How would you like to experience abundance?* Imagine exactly what you desire. (These are good journaling questions to ponder.)

Did this exercise feel silly? Did you think it was childish to ponder these questions? Maybe the images that came into your mind scared you a bit. Did they feel unreal? POSSIBILITY thinking can get intercepted by REALITY or the date stored in your PROGRAM. Your PROGRAM might remind you what is possible based on the experiences you've previously lived or heard about. Were you guided back to imagining a more "realistic" outcome?

To transform your body you must employ POSSIBILITY thinking, no matter what your PROGRAM tries to tell you.

Anything is possible.

POSSIBILITY thinking taps into Infinite Potentials. You can represent the concept of Infinite Potential by names as: The SOURCE, ONE MIND, SPIRIT, ENERGY. If these concepts don't vibe for you, substitute UNIVERSE or LOVE or ALLNESS.

You can access your POSSIBILITY mind by using detailed, palpable visualizations. IMAGINE your desired result. Use declarative prayer or affirmation. Picture yourself connected to your desired outcome. You don't need to be a kid nor do you need to belong to a certain spiritual group to make use of POSSIBILITY mind. You already use POSSIBILITY mind.

Imagine a freak accident. A child's foot is pressed under a car tire. In reaction, the mother, who does not regularly exercise, musters the strength to lift the vehicle off her kid's foot. She lifts a supremely heavy object without any help and without getting injured.

Where did her strength come from? It came from her superconscious vision. It came from an intention to keep her child from being harmed. She was able to summon behavior that matched her desired goal.

She did not hold a competitive thought. She aligned with one pure decision. She chose one option from Infinite Potential or infinite POSSIBILITY: *save my kid*. She did not defer to her established PROGRAM to justify her level or ability or her choice.

POSSIBILITY thinking is choosing
a desired VISION
with
no competing thought, or vision, or belief.

Here's a list of my favorite books that explore the power of the creative mind.

AS A MAN THINKETH, James Allen   1903
THE GAME OF LIFE AND HOW TO PLAY IT, Florence Scovel Shinn 1925
The POWER OF AWARENESS, Neville Goddard 1952
UNLIMITED POWER, Anthony Robbins   1987
The POWERMIND SYSTEM, Michael Monroe Kiefer   1995
POWER VS. FORCE, Dr David Hawkins   1995
The POWER OF INTENTION, Dr Wayne Dyer   2004
THE BIOLOGY OF BELIEF, Bruce Lipton   2005
THE BIG LEAP, Gay Hendricks   2009
BREAKING THE HABIT OF BEING YOURSELF, Joe Dispenza 2012
WISHES FULFILLED, Dr Wayne Dyer   2012

Introducing the 8 healthy habits for her happy life

The RiTual

1. Set meaningful feeling goals every 8-12 weeks + practice
the POST and reward yourself for your progress

2. Practice daily lovetruths

3. Advance-schedule your weekly workouts
and Fuel

4. Exercise for 45-90 minutes 4-6 days every week

5. Balance your Body of Exercise
with cardio, strength training, flexibility, and relaxation

6. Fuel every 4-5 hours and consume half your bodyweight
in ounces of water daily

7. Eat 1-2 cheat meals per week
{no bigger than a hand-size portion—with the thumb up}

8. Sleep between 6-9 hours 6+ nights a week
Go to sleep and wake up at the same times each day

You could leap over the rainbow with these 8 habits right now. I've seen many-a-student dash off with Usain Bolt eagerness to lose 30 pounds. There's nothing I can do to stop you except caution you to slowdown. Pace yourself. Slow and steady will yield favorable, long-lasting results.

Plus, you've got some undercover work to do, first:
De-clutter your mind.
Sift through your mind.
Find limiting thoughts and beliefs, and put them in the dump.

h.**a**.b.i.t

abandon your barriers

Confronting your limiting belief patterns is just as important as setting your meaningful goals.

THE DUMP

I would have never been able to transform my body without a pen, paper, and my imagination. Journaling let me see what was holding me back from my desires. Journaling helped me understand my creative mind.

You have over 50,000 thoughts every day, and many of them are responsible for your beliefs and daily behaviors.

How will you examine the thoughts that are guiding you every day?

Talking helps, however you can hardly remember what you've said 10 minutes after the words leave your mouth. When you journal, you freeze your words on the page. You can return to them and re-view them. The journal lets you witness how your thoughts contribute to your choices.

Saving yourself on your journal pages shows you who you've been. It gives you a space where you can decide and declare who you intend to be.

Get a pencil or pen.
Let's visit The DUMP.

• • •

80% of success is psychology and 20% is mechanics.
Tony Robbins, Life and Business Strategist,
and one of my giant master teachers

Use the journal prompts throughout the book to unpack your thoughts, feelings, and beliefs about your self, your body, and your weight-loss desires. The companion, CAMP OUT WITH THE LEAN HAPPY HEALTHY YOU JOURNAL, contains these questions and more.

LEAN HAPPY HEALTHY YOU Journal

Predict how your BOD will look in 5 years if your lifestyle habits don't change.
Predict your health and self esteem in 10 years

if you don't change anything?

How might your life change when you lose 10 lbs of fat?

Have you ever lost weight and gained it or more back?

How did it feel?

What are you most afraid of experiencing during fat-loss?

What are you uncomfortable about releasing or adding to

your life in order to lose the fat?

(Consider your schedule, groceries, entertainment, activities,

roles, issues, and confidence.)

How will implementing a healthy lifestyle affect your

relationships/friendships? (Positively and negatively)

Recall 4 specific memories when your body image or

health issues caused you emotional pain. Who was there,

what was said, how did you feel? What beliefs did you

form from those experiences?

Recall a time when your body brought you great joy.

Describe.

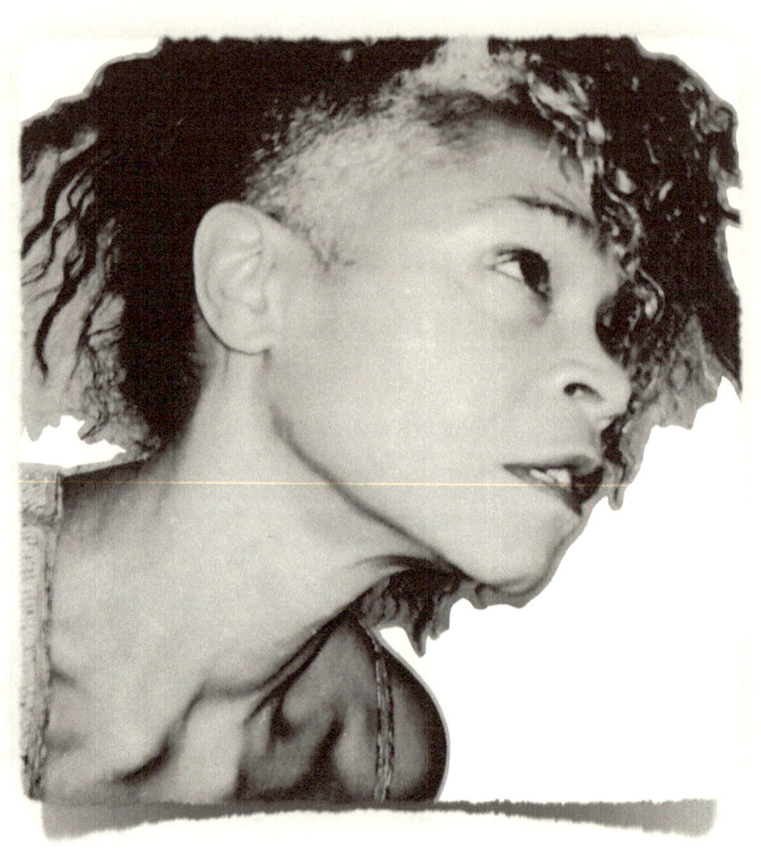

PART THREE

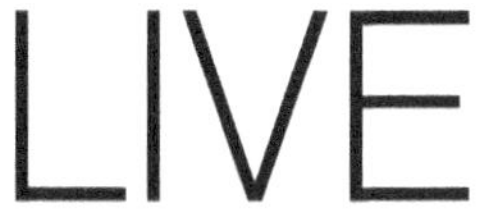

LIVE

ROCK *The RiTual*

1. Set meaningful feeling goals every 8-12 weeks + practice
the POST and reward yourself for your progress

2. Practice lovetruths

3. Advance-schedule your workouts and Fuel

4. Exercise for 45-90 minutes 4-6 days every week

5. Balance your Body of Exercise
with cardio, strength training, flexibility, and relaxation

6. Fuel every 4-5 hours and consume at least half your
bodyweight in ounces of water

7. Eat 1-2 cheat meals per week
{no bigger than a hand-size portion—with the thumb up}

8. Sleep a regulated 6-9 hours 6+ nights of the week

Sustained fat-loss and a healthy lifestyle is a result of practicing
healthy habits of mind, heart, and body.

Healthy habits for your mind.

h.a.**b**.i.t.

bring a desired feeling and vision into your body

Habit #1 Set meaningful feeling goals every 8 -12 weeks. Practice the POST. Celebrate your progress. Reward yourself.

- I want to lose body fat.
- I want to improve my health.
- I want to be happy.

You could toss a penny for each of these generic goals. Plop. Plop. Plop. Now what?

These desires are non-specific and dull. Put wheels on your goals if you want to travel past where you are now. Set goals that raise your pulse and make you wanna holler. Set goals that make you come alive or you won't be inspired longer than it takes to say 1, 2, 3.

Set *get up and go goals*, goals that matter to you.

I want to lose weight. This statement—Meh. *Wanting* won't necessarily get you to move. I want $10,000,000. You? Does wanting 10 million bucks make you determined to go after it? Or does it make you aware that you don't have it? A goal like *I want to lose weight* could be accomplished by losing 1/2 a pound. Get specific.

I want to improve my health.
Why? How would your life change if your health improved? How would improved health affect the people you're around every day? The answers to these questions will help you personalize your goal and make it meaningful.

I want to be happy.
Define your idea of happiness? Have you felt long-term happiness before? In what ways would changing your

body and health unlock happiness? Your answers will help you describe your meaningful goal.

Revisit THE DUMP. Derive meaningful goals from your journaling responses. Set goals that motivate you to *get up and go* toward your vision.

Set meaningful goals by describing, in detail, how you desire to feel. Journal about how you DO NOT want to feel anymore, also. If you remember my story, feeling disgusted and fed-up motivated me to *get up and go* toward my desired transformation.

How might your life be affected if your health did not improve?

Debra.
The doctor said I'm a pre-diabetic. She says if I don't start exercising and lose weight, I'll have to take medication every day. I already take meds for high blood pressure and sleep apnea. I rarely get a full night of sleep.
If my health doesn't improve, I'm gonna be a slave to the pharmacy. I'm afraid of the side effects from taking so many pills. I don't want to be a sick, tired person when I retire in 7 years.

Knowing these things about my health makes me anxious, which I'm sure is not healthy either. I really want to drop 10 pounds this year. I want to lower my blood sugars. Maybe it'll help the snoring. My husband will appreciate that.

Debra has a fear of becoming dependent upon several medications. She's worried about the side effects and illness after retirement. Prescription refills and doctor's visits after retirement could interfere with her goals to travel. The snoring is a burden on her relationship. Getting inadequate sleep leaves her exhausted.

What can Debra do?
First, she must consciously replay these unwanted situations until they feel unbearable. Then she must visualize one, two, or maybe ZERO bottles of pills at her bedside. She could imagine a stack of her favorite books on her bedside table in their place. She must imagine sleeping soundly in a quiet room.

She can vividly imagine and journal about where she would travel after retiring. She can think about how often she would take trips? She must imagine how it would feel to plan each vacation knowing she doesn't have to worry about her health the way she used to. These are real possibilities for Debra if she changes her habits of mind, heart, and body.

Debra's meaningful goals will focus on **two short-term outcomes (feelings) and one long-term body vision.** She can describe how she *expects* to **feel** and how her life will change because of a healthy ritual.

Your turn. Perhaps you want to get fit and healthy because you want to feel confident wearing a halter dress and a two-piece bathing suit. You want to feel energized when you help your daughter move into her first apartment. You want to feel comfortable after a meal instead of sleepy and bloated. When you travel to Spain this summer, you want to walk the cobblestone streets without having to soak your ankles at the end of the day.

How do you desire to feel? What do you desire to experience? How do you expect to feel after practicing *The RiT* for 12 weeks and thereafter? What are your meaningful feeling goals?

Start by identifying how you do not want to feel anymore.

Outline how you <u>do not</u> want to feel anymore
then describe how/what you'd prefer to feel instead.

I don't want to feel or experience... anymore.	Instead, I desire to feel and experience...

CHECK IN

Your goals matter.

Imagine how you desire to feel. Focus on this feeling. Describe how this feeling would "look" in your life.

Knowing how you do not want to feel anymore will help you clarify what you want.

CAMP OUT

Habit #1 <u>Set meaningful feeling goals every</u> <u>8 -12 weeks based on how you want to feel</u> <u>and what you desire to experience</u>

Concentrate on two short-term meaningful feeling goals every 8-12 weeks and one long-term vision every six months.

Describe *what this feeling looks like in your life.* **Make your description personal, detailed, and specific to your life experience.**

Clarifying how you desire to feel will motivate you to *get up and go* toward your goal.

Choose 2 feeling goals from this list or select your own.

powerful	strong	dedicated
motivated	sensual	devoted
fearless	organized	cherished
courageous	purposeful	ambitious
unwavering	committed	enlivened
calm	attractive	confident
energetic	gorgeous	disciplined
focused	decisive	harmonious
positive	centered	sexy

Describe your short-term meaningful feelings.
Use your journal for more space.

I desire to feel_______________over the next 12 weeks.
How will this feeling affect your life? What does this
feeling look like in your life experience? Be specific.
Personalize it.

____

____

____

____

____

____

____

____

____

____

____

____

____

I desire to feel________________over the next 12 weeks.
How will this feeling affect your life? What does this
feeling look like in your life experience? Be specific.
Personalize it.

____

____

____

____

____

____

____

____

____

____

____

*"Get up, Donna. We need to get to the gym before 6:30
or we'll never make it to work on time,"* the PRINCIPLE
mind grumbles. This starts the typical morning
negotiation.

*"Except, you know, we could do a workout this weekend
and stay in bed for another twenty minutes..."*
The PRINCIPLE mind adds a competitive thought. It's not
aligned with Donna's meaningful feeling goal.

Her PRINCIPLE mind remembers that Donna wants to
feel decisive and powerful. *No. Let's do the workout
now. Get up, Donna!*

This mental bargaining goes on for another five minutes.
Donna fumbles out of bed with just enough time to make
it to her 6:30 am kickboxing class.

Have you ever had a morning like Donna's? She made it
to her workout—this time. But her chatty mind put her
decision on trial. One of these mornings Donna will hit
the snooze three more times when her old PROGRAM
wins *rock, paper, scissors* over her willpower.

**Like Donna, you need more than only a <u>meaningful
feeling</u> to keep you focused.**

You need a VISION.

When I got serious about transforming my body, I had to focus on my VISION whenever my willpower got into a catfight with doubt.

I already told you about my habit of visioning, but it bears repeating. I had been journaling and visualizing when I was a child. It worked to bring my goals into reality, so why not try it with my body.

When the students cleared out of the studio after Anna's classes, I'd stand close to the big mirrors. I'd examine my shoulders, turn to the side and check my triceps, then face forward and scan my thighs. I didn't see the body that actually appeared in the mirror. **I visualized what I wanted to see. I saw sculpted arms, shoulders, and legs.**

Imagining my goal as fulfilled changed my held perspective during the journey. I loved the aerobic dance classes. Being able to keep up with Anna was a win for me. I enjoyed watching my body become flexible and exert force. I was so intrigued by the small wins, I stopped rushing my weight-loss process.

My negative self-concept faded. I saw what I loved in
that mirror, I mean I loved what I saw—both. When my
perspective and my beliefs changed to match my
VISION, my body changed.

WRITE A LONG-TERM BODY VISION

**Imagine how you expect to look and feel, and describe
what you expect to experience in 6 months.**

Describe in detail—your health, stamina, energy level, etc.
*How will you look, dress, and feel? What kinds of
compliments will you receive? What will your doctor say?
How will your confidence improve? What types of
activities will you explore?*

Write a BODY VISION every 6 months.

**Your two short-term feeling words and your long-term
BODY VISION are your meaningful goals.** In HABIT #2,
you'll lift your goals and this vision off the page and put
them into your body.

This next part'll help.

PRACTICE THE POST

Your creative mind has a natural tendency to keep familiar PROGRAMS buoyant. Occupy your POSSIBILITY mind with a VISION of what you desire.

Both the PROGRAM and POSSIBILITY minds respond to images and feelings more than words.

POST visual examples of your meaningful feeling goals and body vision. Use pictures, photos, and magazine clippings. **Make a vision board.**

POST your vision board on the refrigerator, in your locker, in your wallet, as your homepage on all your devices; any place where you can see it every day.

TIME FLIES WHEN THE GOALS DRY UP

According to Tony Robbins, *growth* is one of your core human needs. Growth provides the rungs that scale to self-actualization.

A life without growth is outright uninspiring. Without growth, folks interpret time as flying. Their life feels like it's evaporating. Each day gets morphed into the next, forming a blur of Fridays. Another year passes and all one remember was who won the Super Bowl.

Charting your progress will bring your life into consciousness. Your time will become valuable and you'll account for how you spend it.

Though you'll have small wins before the big wins, underscore your small wins along the way. The small wins are happy returns.

At the end of each week, instead of logging your weight on a scale, log your progress points.

Use this checklist.

Each week put a ✓ check where you've made progress!

I feel/have/do MORE...

__endurance

__flexibility

__strength

__agility

__focus

__pleasure

__clarity

__consistency

__energy

__power

__excitement

__desired shape

__comfort

__alignment

__confidence

__desired clothes size

__positive self-talk

__relaxed

__conscious eating

__more self-care (baths,

massages, quiet time...)

__meditation

__adherence to The RiT

__healthy community

__quality rest

__reduction of

"undesirable" food

__healthy recipes and

grocery choices

add your own

You can also write about small wins in your journal.

HAPPY HANGOUTS

Celebrate your big wins. When you achieve your long-term vision, reward yourself with a HAPPY HANGOUT.

A HAPPY HANGOUT is a date with your healthy self
(others can join you).

Suggestions for HAPPY HANGOUTs include:

- one hour massage

- manicure

- pedicure

- new hair color

- movie tickets

- theatre tickets

- healthy cooking class

- buy hobby materials like yarn, paints, scrapbook papers

- a day at the beach

- a Yoga retreat in Costa Rica

- special Yoga class

- personal training sessions

- a new bicycle

- buy sneakers and break them in

- shop for a picture frame to hold a snapshot of the *new you*

Generally, limit edible HAPPY HANGOUT rewards unless
it's a healthy cooking class.

CHECK-IN

Focus on your desired outcome and the feelings associated with it.

POST a written and a visual representation of your meaningful feeling goals and vision where you can review them every day.

Log your progress points weekly.

Celebrate your long-term body vision with a HAPPY HANGOUT!

CAMP OUT

PRACTICE THE HABIT

Habit #1 Reward yourself every 6 months

How will you spend your HAPPY HANGOUT?
Advance-schedule it.

My HAPPY HANGOUT is

____

I'm going to celebrate my HAPPY HANGOUT on
_________________________________ (day + date)

Practice a HAPPY HANGOUT every 6 months at
minimum. Once **The RiT** becomes your natural lifestyle,
you'll find it easier to trust your vision. Self-trust will give
you the fortitude to keep moving.

Healthy habits for your heart.

• • •

Don't let the noise of other's opinions drown out your
own inner voice. And most important, have the courage
to follow your heart and intuition.

They somehow already know what you truly want to
become.

Everything else is secondary.

the historic visionary, Steve Jobs

Habit #2   Practice lovetruths. Bond your desire to your body.

Your heart is a muscle that not only circulates oxygen through your body, it has the power to energize your life. Your heart isn't assertive like your mind. It whispers what you yearn for without sanding the scary parts away or qualifying you to be worthy to receive your requests.

Your heart makes your New Year's resolutions. Your heart makes your birthday wishes. When your heart is fulfilled, you experience a lightness, an openness, joy.

Your heart cannot lie. It's a natural truth-teller. If you listened to your heart more often (and your mind less often) you'd be able to eclipse mental monsters like procrastination, low confidence, and self-loathing. It can be difficult to follow your heart's desire, because you can't always hear it over your PROGRAM. Louder, more forceful beliefs about what's possible rise like firecrackers from your PROGRAM.

When your heart makes a dream request, a feeling pops into your body, then it softens. That's intuition.

Whenever you wish for a goal, the PRINCIPLE mind rushes in to trim your request to fit "your reality". Your reality is informed by the beliefs you've stored in your PROGRAM.

Your PRINCIPLE might reason,

- *"Ah. Hold on, sistah. You can't earn $200,000 a year. You didn't finish college. What are you going to tell them in the interview when they ask about your level of education?"*
- *"Ease up, cowgirl! You'll never be able to pay a 30-year mortgage at your age. Be happy you have a roof over your head. You live in a nice apartment now—nicer than the one you grew up in. Aren't you satisfied with that?"*
- *"Calm down. Not everybody is gonna meet a partner they can marry! You know how hard it is to find a good partner these days, anyhow. At least you have good friends."*
- *"How do you expect to raise a child on your own? You need a partner to do that kind of thing. It wouldn't be fair for the kid—not having two parents at home. Be happy you have a dog. That's enough of a responsibility to manage."*

If your heart's desire is to earn a $200,000 salary, own a 3-bedroom house, be loved by a partner who thinks you're amazing, raise a child on your own, run a half marathon by next year, wear a size 8 pant, develop ripped abs, and feel confident wearing a tangerine striped bikini when you're 55, you can do it. Desire it now, with all your heart.

HEART-CENTERED WHAT?

Your body responds to your most prevalent thoughts and feelings. Your positive vibes (energy) and affirmative messages strengthen your body. They can heal your body, too. Heart-centered emotions strengthen and heal you, too.

Have you ever attended a class, concert, or church session that made you feel inspired or up-lifted? Recall the sensation in your body. Was it a feeling of lightness? Increased physical energy? A feeling of mental clarity? An overall sense of freedom? You'd probably describe the experience as timeless, expansive, and joyful.

When heart-centered or heart-dominated energy circulates through your body, your mental function is alleviated from its critical, judgmental, protective nature to optimistic and encouraged.

Whenever you feel inspired and joyful your body produces endorphins, happy hormones, that give rise to a euphoric sensation. Endorphins reduce pain and improve your immune response. Serotonin levels increase. Serotonin can reduce your appetite and halt cravings. Dopamine increases which sharpens your concentration.

Imagine a time when you've felt frustrated, angered, or depressed by a challenge. Imagine an experience that made you want to hide, shrink, or sleep till the feeling passed. During this time, you might pray or bury your head in a pillow and cry to get through the feeling. Let's say that you choose to weep or pray or commune with nature to discharge your negative feelings. Crying, praying, and communing with nature are life-giving, heart-centered ways to neutralize difficult feelings.

GET INTO THE GROOVE

When you **regularly** feel *inspired* and when you maintain heart-felt *joyful* feelings, the brain's neural networks carve an *inspired* groove that **records a memory of**

INSPIRATION. If you feel *inspired* often, your *inspiration* groove deepens. **If you often seek to feel *inspired* your brain becomes addicted to feeling *inspired.* Unconsciously, you'll seek ways to feel this way again and again.** *Neuroplasticity* is the malleable nature of your brain to form, memorize, and replay thinking and feeling patterns until they become habits of thinking.

When you use healing modalities like prayer, affirmation, nature, deep breathing, tears, or other healing modalities to neutralize the difficult emotions like frustration, anger, and anxiety, you are also making a heart-centered choice. *Connection, courage, acceptance, gratitude, forgiveness,* and *love* are heart-centered energetics. They reduce the stress response and relax your blood pressure. They also wire your brain by carving grooves of *connection, acceptance, gratitude* into your mental memory. If you often choose *connection, acceptance,* and *gratitude* to deal with challenges, your brain will form a habit of feeling these emotions whenever you have challenges or pain. Once again, these heart-centered choices have a positive affect on your body and your brain.

However, if challenges, difficulties, and pain deploy you to judge, criticize, and complain excessively and heighten feelings of hate, rage, and fear, you are not making a heart-centered choice. These are mind-centered reactions. They trigger the stress response. Mind-centered energetics produce excessive cortisol and adrenaline. They suppress immunity, cause muscle tightness, impair digestion and proper elimination, and elevate your pulse. Levels of dopamine and serotonin drop, contributing to the risk of depression. The longer or more often you marinate in thoughts and feelings of sadness, helplessness, or despair, while simultaneously feeling rage, aggression, and/or anxiety; your brain's neural pathways will organize mental grooves that PROGRAM these negative feelings. Eventually, these negative feeling grooves will deepen. Feeling bad (and sick) will become something your mind and body will seek. Your brain wires it into a habitual feeling state, which means your body/mind will keep looking for ways to feel like this. Yucko.

How are you wiring your brain?

WOO WOO

Your heart is a messenger. It has something important to tell you. The heart forms before the brain in utero. The heart sends more information up to the brain about how you feel than it receives from the brain.

Heart-centered energetics are being studied at the HeartMath Institute in Boulder Creek, CA. An EKG measures your heart's electrical wave. According to the HeartMath Institute, you have a 360 degree magnetic field that emanates 4-8 feet from your heart. This field is a bandwidth of energy, similar to a radio wave. A **coherent** electromagnetic field of heart-centered energy emits a vibration of love, compassion, acceptance, joy, hope, gratitude, and the like. Feelings of rage, grief, depression, and fear create an **incoherent** field around your body. I like to refer to this magnetic field as your *vibration* or your *vibe*.

Time for the *woo woo.*

Your vibe **entrains** or syncs with the strongest energy or *vibe* around it. In other words, the energy from your heart can either match or elevate the energy around you. This is referred to as entrainment.

Imagine a room with two pianos. When you play middle C on one piano, the other piano automatically vibrates the middle C tone, even though no one has tapped the key. The second piano entrained with the first piano.

Since your body entrains to the energy around you, how do you suppose your social environment affects your confidence or your ability to lose weight?

Finding a tribe that shares your vibe is absolutely necessary. More on that at the end of this book. For now, be aware that your body entrains to your vibe and the energy around it.

YOUR VIBE

The late Japanese scientist, Dr. Masura Emoto, conducted a experiment to observe how intentions change water. He taped feeling words on clear jars of water and froze them. Emoto photographed the crystals the next day. The jars with words like *HAPPINESS, THANK YOU,* and *LOVE* taped on them had well formed, symmetric crystals that glowed like radiant snowflakes in the photos. The water crystals that were asymmetric, murky, and dull came from the jars with words like *YOU MAKE ME SICK and HATE* taped on them. Also, polluted water from a Japanese stream showed the same asymmetric, muddled pattern. He rephotographed the polluted water after a Buddhist monk prayed over it, and the prayed-over crystals changed into symmetric, glowing snowflake-like crystals. *LOVE* and *GRATITUDE* beautified the water crystals the most. Dr. Emoto's experiment suggests that loving, grateful feelings and intentions can positively alter water molecules.

Your body is more than 70% water. Will a self-loathing mental energy morph your body to match? Can positive self-talk heal you? I'm sure it can.

The lovetruth practice, visualizing the body and life you desire, will raise your vibe. Practicing this habit might feel intimidating at first, especially if you have difficulty seeing your body differently from what reality presents. However, it's possible to hold a vision of something you've never experienced before.

Dr. Martin Luther King Jr declared A DREAM (a vision) on the steps of the Lincoln Memorial.

It is a dream deeply rooted in the American dream.
I have a dream that one day this nation will rise up, live
out the true meaning of its creed: 'We hold these truths
to be self-evident, that all men are created equal.'

He declared a new way of life for Americans, detailing
freedoms that had never been experienced before.
King's devotion to his dream sparked emotional
coherence throughout the crowd of listeners, present and
otherwise. He declared something no one had never
seen in their reality, however his emphasis on love and
connection gave his dream the power to mobilize the
American spirit. His energy and intention entrained
America.

When actor Jim Carrey was broke and struggling in
Hollywood, he wrote himself a check for $10,000,000.
He post-dated the "paycheck" for Thanksgiving 1995
and kept it in his wallet. For years, he'd sit on a hill near
Mulholland Drive in L.A. holding the crumpled check
while imagining himself working gigs that paid
$10,000,000. He'd imagine collaborating with top
directors and receiving praise and awards. He'd stay on
the hill until his vision felt real. He imagined his vision
whenever he auditioned or worked on small jobs in
Hollywood. Jim Carrey was cast and paid $10,000,000
for the movie *Dumb and Dumber* in 1995, the exact year
he'd put on the check.

Jim Carrey was poor when he began entraining to his
request. He'd never earned large amounts of money

before, yet he was able to **see and feel** and *get up and go* toward his goal until it became his reality. He projected himself into what he loved. He felt grateful for reaching his goal way before it actually happened. This is POSSIBILITY thinking, entrainment, and heart-centered coherence.

You can come from impoverishment and build a life of abundance and wealth. If you achieved a 2.0 grade-point average in high school you can create a six-figure business by age 30 doing what you love. You can be 70 lbs overweight for 15 years and lose 80 lbs in a year and keep it off! Your past does not matter when you harness your creative mind, visualize what you love, and *get up and go* toward your meaningful goal. Believe your desire is possible.

CHECK IN

Your body bonds with your thoughts and emotions. Heart-centered emotions like *LOVE, APPRECIATION, COMPASSION,* and *JOY* energize and regulate your bodily systems. Mind-centered emotions like *fear, rage, depression,* and *anxiety* constrict your bodily systems. Mind-centered emotions felt in excess can make you sick. Heart-centered emotions can entrain you to a heart-centered life experience.

The lovetruth practice lets you visualize and declare your meaningful feeling goals. Repeating the lovetruth visualization daily will bond you to the outcome.

You can visualize having, being, and doing something you've never had, been, or done before.

Your imagination can penetrate life.

• • •

Just believe in yourself. Even if you don't, pretend you
do and at some point you will.

Serena Williams,
who shows All Things are Possible with practice,
unwavering focus, and belief

CAMP OUT

PRACTICE THE HABIT

Habit #2 Practice lovetruths

First, re-view your meaningful feeling words and your journal entry about how you desire to experience those feelings.

WRITE two lovetruth declarations for your next 8-12 weeks based on your meaningful feeling entries.

Simply sum up your meaningful feeling entries into 1-3 sentences.

Here are the GUIDELINES for each lovetruth declaration:

1. Lovetruths are specific, descriptive, and personal. **Use *I* and *My* to personalize them. Describe them so you can see them clearly, like they're real.**

Meaningful feeling word = *energized*

Non-specific, general example: **I have more energy.**

Example of a specific and personal example based on your journal entry: **I have the energy to swim in my own lane for an hour. My son and I swim every Saturday morning at the community center during his swim season. Because I work late during the week, our Saturday swims have improved our relationship. After swimming we stop at the farmer's market, then go home and make breakfast together.**

2. Declare them in present tense. Assume your lovetruth has already happened.
Use the words: **I am, My, I have, I feel, I experience, I see,** and **I enjoy.**

Meaningful feeling word = *sexy*

Don't write a wish for the future: **I hope to fit into a sexy dress for my cousin's wedding.**

Write something like this declaration in present tense:
My back is exposed. The dress is strapless. Debra chose magenta for the bridesmaids. The color looks good against my skin. My waist is as small as it was when I got married, which is simply amazing. My husband says I look like the bride.

<u>Meaningful feeling word = *cherished*</u>

Write something like this declaration in present tense: **I'm enjoying the classes after work. I made three new friends from the boxing class on Tuesdays and Thursdays. They keep reminding me how far I've come and cheer for me when I hit the speed bag.**

Ready to write yours?

Write two lovetruths.

Use the words : *I am, My, I have, I feel, I experience, I see, I enjoy...*

1

2

Now practice the lovetruth visualization, also called a POSSIBILITY PRACTICE, and imagine the details of your meaningful feelings.

For your **lovetruth practice—**

• Read your lovetruths a few times then sit for the breathing practice.

- The breathing practice and body relaxation may last 2–4 minutes.
- The visualization may last 1–3 minutes.

Imagine your lovetruth in detail.
Your mind is influenced by imagery and feeling.

Here is a lovetruth visualization.

CENTERING

Sit on the floor or in a firm chair. Cross or extend your
legs. Keep your torso upright yet relaxed.
You may close your eyes.
Breathe slowly.
Take an easy breath in through the nostrils, exhale
through the mouth. Repeat one more time. Exhale silently
or with sound like a sigh.
Continue nostril breathing. Inhale through the nostrils,
slowly exhale through the nostrils.
As you breathe, notice your fingers relaxing. Your knees
and ankles relax. Your breath becomes slower. Notice
your mouth relax. The space around your eyes relax.
Your mind relaxes.

VISUALIZATION

Say one of your meaningful feeling words silently in your
mind. Feel it in your body.
Notice how you experience the word.
What image does it conjure?
What other desirable feelings does it inspire?
See yourself experiencing this lovetruth like it's real.

IMAGINE the other meaningful feeling word.
IMAGINE its corresponding lovetruth.
See yourself experiencing this lovetruth like it's real.
What do you notice/feel?
Experience your lovetruth with all your senses.

To close, take three deep nostril breaths.
Exhale them slowly.
Place your palms together at your heart's center and
bow to POSSIBILITY. Say THANK YOU, NAMASTE, or
any word or phrase that honors your belief.

Imagine your lovetruths at least once a day:

* upon rising in the morning
* during Cardio training (if you're practicing cardio alone)
* after your workout while you stretch
* in the shower (the POSSIBILITY practice)
* before bed

Imagine your lovetruths at the same time of day every week.

Practice the POST. Post your lovetruths in a central station and keep them in your journal. Look at them every day.

• • •

It's the repetition of affirmations that leads to belief.
And once that belief becomes a deep conviction,
things begin to happen.
Muhammad Ali, The Greatest,
who showed us how powerful words can be

h. a. b. **i.** t.

initiate a series of behaviors

that align with your vision

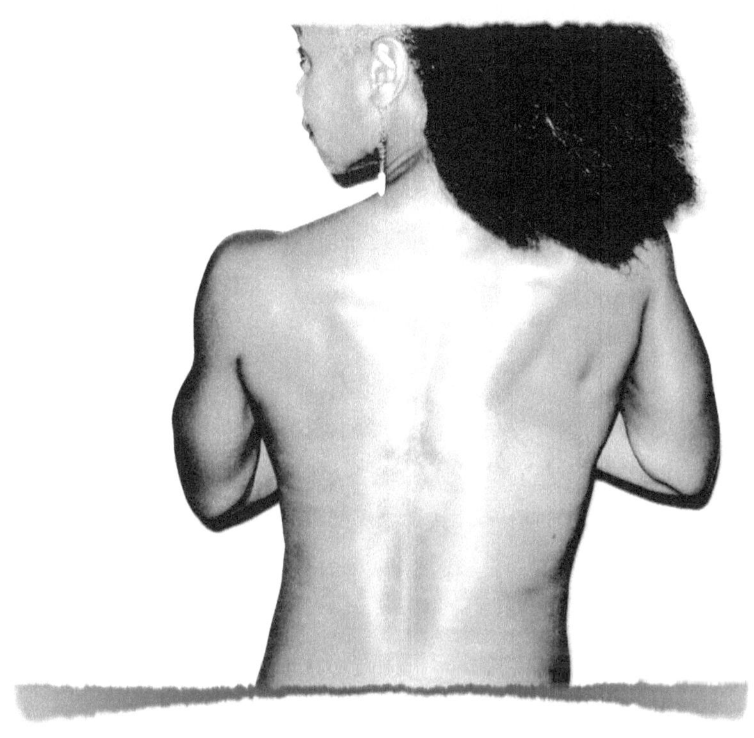

Healthy habits

for

your body.

• • •

Let's get serious about our days and what we are
becoming because of them.

Let's get serious about the aim and enjoyment of a
meaningful life. It is time to value the hour once more
and refuse to give up our lives to the distractions and
nonsense.

It is time to make our own way and get back to our day.

For this we declare: We Shall Reclaim Our Agenda.

HABIT # 3

ADVANCE-SCHEDULE your workouts and your fuel

When will you schedule your workouts?

Are you thinking about it now? Good. Write your workout schedule. Double-good! Don't let a slight gust of emotional wind blow your house of goals out of reach. Erect boundaries around this workout schedule. Uphold it as sacred.

In softball you're supposed to hit the ball and run like lightning to first base. You're encouraged to over-run first base. Your called "safe" after you tap the base, so you can charge at first base with all your might. However, if you over-run second or third base you could get tagged "out". For the other bases prepare to slide or check the field to see if it's safe to run.

RUN LIKE LIGHTNING EVERY WEEK

Perhaps you'll begin using the 8 habits of *The RiT* the way you'd run to first base, charged with excitement and high hopes. Maybe you'll run at your fat-loss goals with lightning speed. But after a few weeks you hesitate and check the field of your random feelings before you run toward your goal.

Stay focused once you pass your first successful weeks of *The RiT.* Be mindful not to fall back into random decision-making. Do not consult your fluctuating feelings to decide whether to exercise.

You've chosen a couple dominant feelings, your meaningful feelings. Move toward those.

At the beginning of each week, advance-schedule your workouts and follow that schedule.

**Conserve effort by following
the same workout schedule each week.**

Give a *heads up* to the people who spend time with you. Tell them when you'll be working out (busy). You'll command respect for your non-negotiable commitment.

I know, I know. Life's not all mermaids and unicorns. Your schedule is sure to meet with opposition. Two challengers who threaten your workout schedule are the OPAs and OPOs: Other People's Agendas and Other People's Opinions about you, your program, your new habits, your new thoughts, the specificity of your goals, and your vision.

You've arranged to go to a Sunday morning Pilates class only to awaken to an unexpected invitation to do something rather not decline? You get a text from the person you've been stalking for a while on Facebook. The person asks you to meet for brunch. *Well, yeah!*

After a couple text exchanges ending with *meet-cha at noon*, you prepare the tub for a luxurious bubble soak. You set your hair, douse your back and bra in Chanel no 5, try-on four different pairs of slacks, then meet the cutie at the restaurant by 12:03. NNNNN! That's the sound of a wrong-decision buzzer. You've skipped your Pilates class—again.

You could have had it all. You could have happily hummed SADE tunes during a quick shower after the Pilates workout. You could've stuck with the first pair of slacks as they would've buttoned-up nicely after the challenging ab workout. Plus, you would've felt guiltless about sharing flan with your brunch darling.

Your workout schedule is sacred. The people who care about you will understand this. If they don't, train them.

You'll be pleased with yourself if you show them what to expect from you.

Your agenda matters more than Other People's Agendas. Advance-schedule each week's workouts and **attend them as scheduled**.

The OPOs (Other People's Opinions) may try to persuade you to trash your plans.

Liz asked her best friend, Dani, to help her find a new desk and chair from IKEA Saturday morning. Dani loved shopping at IKEA. She said she'd be ready to go by 11:30 am. Liz suggested they get to the store before 11. Dani apologized, "Oh Liz, my spinning class isn't over till 10:30. I'll take a quick shower and rush to your place by 11:30. Promise!"

Liz was disappointed. "Can't you skip spinning this week? Haven't you been going to the gym too much anyway? Don't you think you need a break? I really want to get to the store early."

Dani didn't know what to say. She advance-scheduled 4 workouts for the week. She was used to doing 5 workouts, but had to cancel one to attend a work function on Thursday. This would mean missing another workout. She wanted to help Liz. She was conflicted.

OPOs will show up whether you're ambivalent or deeply committed to your goals.

Julia shared an apartment with her sister and best friend, Jennifer. Both sisters desired to lose weight since junior high school. Over the years they tried many diets together. Usually the positive results would disappear around the holidays.

Julia started practicing **The RiTual** *in September. By November 12, she'd gone from 195 lbs down to 172 lbs. In order to lose an average of 2 lbs a week, Julia advance-scheduled 4 fitness classes every week. Julia also hired a personal trainer for Sundays.*

One particular Sunday, Jennifer seemed irritated at Julia. Julia arrived home 20 minutes later than she promised for dinner. She refused to put gravy or cornbread on her plate.

"Yeah, we'll see how long that lasts," Jennifer cut her eyes at Julia then made herself a plate of food.

"Jenn, you know it's not personal. I love your cooking. I just don't want another set-back this time. I want to lose 12 more pounds by the end of the year."

"Get serious, Julia. You do these crazy programs every year. You already know what'll happen. Right now, you're wide-eyed about getting to the gym. You're eating this

healthy stuff they tell you to eat. I mean, what are you gonna do when you get too busy to workout? What are you gonna do at Thanksgiving—excuse yourself from my turkey and gravy? That's crazy, girl. You're just gonna gain the weight back, like we usually do—remember? Have you thought about that?"

Julia felt sick.

OPOs. When I first lost a significant amount of weight following my consistent workout schedule, someone close to my heart cornered me with the same kinds of questions in a doubtful tone. I responded, "I WON'T GAIN THE WEIGHT BACK. I'M GONNA KEEP IT OFF."

Saying those words strengthened my conviction to live up to them. At first I was panicked over how I'd live up to them. I was terrified about the future. Except that the process that changed my body gave me more discipline and showed me I could trust myself. I figured I'd use the same tools that transformed my mind and body the first time if I faced issues in the future.

You're gonna keep the fat lost, too. You'll have the tools. Plus, you don't have to focus on your schedule next year nor do you need to know how you'll accommodate it next year. You only have to know this week's schedule. You need to know next week's schedule at the beginning of next week, and so on. When life hands you a new schedule, you can update your weekly workouts.

Martin Luther King, Jr. said that after you decide to advance toward something momentous, do not become overwhelmed by *how* you'll climb the entire staircase. **Climb one stair at a time.**

In PART FOUR I'll explain ways to handle interference from your OPOs and OPAs. Though some people in your life won't understand your new healthy lifestyle, some will. I'll explain why you need to find someone who supports you. It'll help you embody your vision.

CHECK-IN

Randomness is on the b-side of indecision. Don't play those records.

Advance-schedule your workouts every week. Great accomplishment is not achieved by the random.

Schedule. Remain consistent.

No matter what.

CAMP OUT

Habit #3 Advance-schedule your workouts each week and advance-schedule your fuel for the day

You can practice habit #3 after you read the next three habits. Start thinking about **where** you'll workout and **what** kinds of workouts interest you.

Release the blocks that limit you from advance-scheduling. Put your goal into your calendar every week.

LEAN HAPPY HEALTHY YOU Journal

List four activities or habits that suck away your time.

What activity could you reduce in order to make time for
your workouts?

Have you encountered OPOs and OPAs regarding your
workouts and health?

What kinds of things do they say to you?
How do they make you feel?

How might you respond to an OPO or OPA that bumps up
against your workout schedule?

Habit #4   EXERCISE for 45 - 90 minutes
4-6 days a week

Do you value your time?

If you spend time befriending Bravo TV's housewives
most days of the week, you might become a well-versed
critic of shady, girlfriend dramas.

If you tell Alexa to snooze five times, instead of rising
early, lacing your sneakers, and keeping your advance-
scheduled workout, you could become a gremlin of guilt
whose only prize is 20 extra minutes of groggy sleep.

Are BRAVO soaps and shallow sleep worth more to you
than burning 300 calories, raising your energy, and
combating stress? Which seems painful to you? Which is
more pleasurable?

Dedicating your valuable time to copious episodes of the
"Housewives of Des Moines", kitten videos on YouTube,
or the corner seat of your sectional for a Mr. Big season
of Law and Order won't burn fat, build muscle, or
improve your self-confidence.

You've got seven days every week, Beyonce. Lose the non-productive, mind-numbing habits if they get in the way of achieving your meaningful goals. Interrupt these time-suckers. Move toward what really matters.

Advance-schedule 4-6 days of exercise every week. Who might you become if you do?

HOT AND HEALTHY MEDICINE

Exercise does more than give you a hot bod. It circulates nutrients to your cells, slows aging, alters your mood (I love that), and improves your sleep. Take your medicine at least 4 times and as often as 6 times a week.

Beyond controlling body fat, there's another major benefit to exercising most days of the week.

Exercise detoxifies you from the harmful effects of stress.

MY STRESS IS TWENTY STORIES HIGH, YOURS IS A MICROPHONE

What makes me feel stressed might not feel stressful to you. I used to sing in front of hundreds of people. The bigger the audience, the better I felt. This might cause you to have a panic attack, ripe with a pulse surge, purple skin, and soaked armpits at the thought of singing in front of two puppies.

However, if you forced me to stand in line for one of those twenty-story, 90 degree dropping rollercoasters at FUN WORLD, I'd lose my breath. My stomach would tangle till I could taste breakfast. My glasses would slip to the side of my sweaty nose. You wouldn't be able to hear me gasping for the drumming from my chest. I do not feel safe or happy on rollercoasters, you see. They raise my level of stress.

If you enjoy fast tin cans that drop, leaving your stomach forty-seconds behind, your body would perceive rollercoasters as exciting. Even if you felt the same physical experiences as I, high heart rate, sweat on your nose, a turbulent stomach—excitement feels similar to anxiety—you'd benefit from a rise in endorphins because of your excitement. I'd become flooded with cortisol because of my fear.

The coaster itself is not stressful. Your perception of the experience determines how your body responds. Your body doesn't need to undergo an actual experience to feel stressed, either. Thinking about a stressor creates the same physical response as experiencing the stressor in real-life.

No one with a pulse can avoid stress. There's nothing you can do to get away from it, unless you retreat to a mountainside cavern in the Himalayas (but then you'd have to deal with bats). Some stressors are good for you. Good stressors can force you off the fence of indecision into action. Good stress can energize you to tackle a task with strength and speed. A stress response can prepare your body to react to danger with urgency, enabling you to fight or flee or freeze.

But, if your perception of stress is rampant in your life, it doesn't bring a happy return to your body or mind. Chronic stress that doesn't dissipate for weeks, months, or longer can make you sad, sick, and fat.

It's raining. You have to walk the dog before work. Your sweet pooch takes more time to sniff out the perfect pee-spot due to the wet sidewalk. You haven't brewed coffee yet. Uh-oh.

Traffic is thicker than usual thanks to the rain, your pup, and other delays like burning your tongue on your coffee. You need to move lanes, but the dude singing in the black Mustang won't let you in. You slam the honk and spit curses into your empty passenger seat. Luckily, you make it to your exit and make it to work only five minutes late.
{Blood pressure spike. Sweaty armpits. Soiled shirt. Mild headache. You need another coffee.}
Scrolls of emails await you. You consider smashing your head onto your keypad, but that could startle your co-workers and jam the keys (like last week). You consider pretending you haven't seen the messages. You could tell folks their emails befell spam.
{Shallow breathing. Elevated heart rate, still. Sharp stomach pangs. Craving candy. You pop a butterscotch, followed by 4 more and proceed to answer emails.}
Lunch time.
There's a fried meat option on the menu. There's pizza. It smells like oregano and sausage. It's free. *God, if I eat this, it'll junk my diet. Maybe one slice... Maybe I'll pull off*

*the pepperoni, the cheese... Maybe I'll eat two pieces
and skip dinner tonight...* {Bloated from three pepperoni
slices. Dehydrated from 4 coffees and, somehow, you're
sleepy.}

During your break, you grab a Venti latte with three
Equals. Starving. You add one mini-bagel with the cream
cheese hidden inside.

The commute home takes twice as long. Your empty
passenger seat is dented by the curse words you've spat
into the leather.

You chew a bag of Doritos in 8 seconds, then pass out
on the couch. It's only 6 pm.

{Low blood sugar. A healthy fat like walnuts or almonds
with berries or a high-fiber carb like a pear or guava fruit
would've fed you better energy—followed by a short
workout, yoga, or walk in nature. A 10-minute nap
would've been fine, not 75 minutes.}

You wake up from your nap, grumpy as a smurf. At 7:15
pm you stick a green, boxed meal into the microwave.
You chew something meaty and saucy, while
simultaneously shuffling through documents for your
presentation tomorrow.

Your phone reads 10 o'clock. Time to walk the dog. You
can't relax until you've checked Facebook and compared
your life to the fabulous lives of friends and people you
don't know (yet friended). By 2 am, you finally pass out,

with your computer screen on. The blue glow makes
your mind spiral into an epicenter of inferior feelings that
push you into dreaming about weird stuff. Throughout
the night your pulse is as high as if you were dancing
Salsa. You wake up exhausted.

When you frequently experience and/or perceive events
in your life as stressful, and when you habitually
consume processed foods or unhealthy fat and sugar in
high quantities, and when you lack adequate sleep or
rest, you become a strong candidate for (DING DING
DING DING) stress overload.

Chronic stress is the main cause of disease and high
body-fat. Chronic stressors cause your adrenal glands to
produce adrenaline, also called epinephrine, which
accelerates your heart rate. Your immune response
weakens. Calcium absorption decreases causing you to
bloat. Uncomfortable, wouldn't you say?

And then there's that hormone, cortisol.

Surely, you've heard of it. It's all the rage. Cortisol is not
a total tyrant. The adrenal glands produce it to help your
body reduce inflammation during a stressful episode.
Imagine the inflammatory response when you're

wounded. The area gets red, swollen, and tender to the touch. The inflammation creates a boundary around the injured area so you won't bother it while it heals. This is the natural inflammatory process.

During chronic stress, the inflammatory response acts as if your whole body is injured. Inflammation largely affects the cells of your organs and muscles instead of a smaller, specific area.

Chronic stress makes your body secrete excessive cortisol. When extra cortisol floods your bloodstream, it disrupts insulin from pushing sugar from your foods into your muscles and organs. Instead, the glucose (sugar) gets rerouted to a different place: your fat cells. The fat cells that cuddle your abdominal organs are especially congenial to the extra glucose. Expanded fat cells equal an expanded belly.

What exactly in this great life could cause you to feel so stressed out? Your mind. Your perceptions. An inability to discharge and neutralize difficult emotions.

Also, if you drink pots of coffee daily, slam Red Bulls, or pop other stimulants, if you check your phone for social media updates or text updates every 5 minutes, eat fast-food, packaged food, and/or processed food regularly; you could be unhinging the floodgates for cortisol and adrenaline to consume your body and enlarge your belly.

To lessen the impact of chronic stress on your system, **you need to exercise**. Also, practicing yoga meditation, writing in your journal, making love, making art, hugging a tree, receiving massage, and laughing—these are a few activities that'll reduce the stress response. They could save your life. They can also be the difference between choosing to wear an oversized hoodie or a silver bikini top on a gorgeous summer night.

Chronic stress ain't no good.

Please consult your healthcare specialist if you experience more than one of these symptoms regularly.

Frequent headaches, sore or stiff neck
Clenched jaw or grinding teeth
Back or muscle spasms
Frequent colds or infections
Frequent allergy attacks
Upset stomach or frequent heartburn
Constipation/diarrhea

Panic attacks or breathing problems
Excessive worry, anxiety, or nervousness (fidgeting)
Frequent rise to anger or hostility
Depression or frequent mood swings (crying outbursts)
A radical change of appetite
Insomnia or sleeping too much
Constant overwhelm
Intense loneliness
Difficulty making decisions, forgetfulness
A loss of care about your appearance
Increased use of alcohol or drugs

These could be symptoms of chronic stress. Ask your health specialist if there are specific exercise guidelines for you to consider. You will benefit from the *lovetruth visualization* and the *mental massage* coming up later.

YOUR STRESS-LESS PILL

Exercise can neutralize the stress response. It can take your mind off your stressor and focus it on your breathing, alignment, and proper form. The endorphins, natural pain-killers, strengthen your immune system and elevate your mood. Your *good mood* can last for hours after your exercise session, sometimes all day.

However, overtraining, working out at extremely high intensities, without interspersing low-intensity workouts or relaxation practices throughout the week, can also put your body under stress.

Incorporate no more than 4 days of high-intensity exercise per week with lower intensity workouts on the other days. Treat your body to a relaxation practice 1-3 days during the week (this is explained in habit #5) or simply schedule 1-3 days of rest from exercise. With proper recovery practices, your body will get stronger and you'll be able to stave off chronic stress, illness, and injury.

High-intensity exercise is defined as any workout that maintains a heart rate between 85-90% of your **heart rate maximum** for 20-minutes or more. You'll learn how to calculate your *exercising heart rate* in the next habit. For now, understand that 85-90% of your maximum heart rate is so intense it's difficult to talk. You can't catch your next breath between words! Cardio workouts like running and sprinting, spinning, kick-boxing, jumping rope, and dancing with fast-moves and jumping sequences are examples of exercising at an intensity that revs your heart rate up, up, and over 85% of your heart rate maximum.

Increase or decrease the intensity of your workout by adjusting the speed, range of motion, position, resistance, resting period, or level of impact.

Refrain from **high intensity or heavy strength training** of the same muscle group (besides abs) on back to back days. Individual muscles, like biceps and triceps, need a day or two of rest between focused strength training sessions to recover, repair, and grow stronger.

Here is an effective 4-day a week exercise program:

Monday : Full-body strength training circuit 45 minutes. stretch for 15 minutes after work [high intensity]
Wednesday : Spinning class after work. Stretch and work abs with intervals of push ups for 20 minutes. [high intensity]
Thursday : Vinyasa Yoga class for 90 minutes after work [high or low intensity]
Saturday : Run 3 miles in 30 minutes on the track in the morning after breakfast then Full-body calisthenics for 15 minutes. After, stretch for 15 minutes [high intensity]

Here are two examples of effective 5-day exercise
programs:

ONE

Tuesday : Kick-boxing class 45 minute. Stretch 15 min.
[high intensity]
Wednesday : Pilates mat class 60 minute [low intensity]
Thursday : African dance class 60 minute. Stretch 10 min.
[high intensity]
Saturday : Full-body strength training circuit
[high or low intensity]
Sunday : Pilates mat class 60 minute. [low intensity]

TWO

Monday : Walk uphill on the treadmill for 30 min.
Upper body strength training 20 min. Stretch 10 min.
[low intensity]
Tuesday : Vinyasa Yoga class in a studio 90 minutes
[high intensity]
Wednesday . Jog 15 min. Lower body strength training
40 min. Stretch 10 min. [low or high intensity]
Friday : Boxing circuit class 45 min. Stretch 10 min.
[high intensity]
Saturday : Full body strength training 40 min. Stretch 15
min. [low or high intensity]

The days off are for resting and muscle-recovery. Incorporate a relaxation practice on off-days. More about relaxation in the next habit.

And here is an effective 6-day exercise program:

Monday : Full-body strength training 60 minutes. [high intensity] Stretch 15 minutes.
Tuesday : Power walk on the treadmill 30 minutes [low intensity, higher intensity the faster you walk and if you use hills] Stretch 15 minutes.
Wednesday : Upper body strength circuit for 30 minutes. Then Pilates for 60 minutes [high or low intensity]
Thursday : Zumba class for 60 minutes [high intensity]
Saturday : Spin class for 45 min. After, 15 minute stretch. [high intensity]
Sunday : Yin Yoga class for 90 minutes [low intensity]

The strength training days are positioned between cardio and Yoga days to let the muscles fully recover. Also, see where the two high intensity cardio classes on Thursday and Saturday have a day between for muscle recovery.

Yoga and Pilates can be considered high intensity workouts, depending on the style, props, and overall sequencing of the postures. Traditional yoga studios schedule classes for 90 minutes to 2 hours.

If yoga is your primary discipline, schedule no more than 4 exercise days of an intense physical practice with a variety of postures that strengthen your whole body. Practice a restorative or Yin style of yoga for muscular recovery 1-3 days a week.

DID YOU HEAR A POP?

Your body is susceptible to injury when it's exposed to intense, repetitive movement patterns of the same ranges of motion, using the same muscle groups. Both injury and stress result from exercises that push the body without proper form, alignment, or regulated breathing.

Camille advance-scheduled 4 miles of running through the park after work 5 days a week. At first she loved her routine. It felt peaceful and effective. It also gave her time to review the day. She used to be an athlete in high school, so her body easily adapted to running. Running melted the excess weight quickly. She dropped 9 lbs during the first month. She added another running day to speed her results.

By the 3rd month her desire to run waned. By the 4th month, she hated running. Hated it. She got headaches on the evenings after she ran. Her right Achilles felt tight when she ran.

Camille tried everything to stomach the feelings of disgust toward running. She downloaded P!NK's greatest hits and invested in new aquamarine sneakers with glow in the dark laces. Still, running felt boring and her right heel began to hurt.

Camille told herself she was not a quitter and if running got the fat off, she was just gonna have to keep rolling her soles. By the end of the month, Camille gave in. Running added too much stress to her life. She skipped her running session on Saturday. By the following Saturday she hadn't run at all.

Problem: Camille enjoyed running, but because she ran 25 days out the month for four months straight, she started feeling the effects of overtraining. She exercised at a high intensity without scheduling recovery practices.

Solution: Camille could have scheduled other forms of cardio exercise like power-walking, biking, or skating. She could have run shorter courses at slower speeds. She needed to program a balanced Body of Exercise to stave off boredom, injury, and stress.

In the next habit, I'll explain why you need to schedule a holistic Body of Exercises that produce strength, stamina, stability, and alignment.

CHECK-IN

Choose a <u>variety</u> of exercise types. <u>Vary exercise
intensities</u> to strengthen your heart, bones, muscles, and
mind, and to prevent injuries. Also, consider modifying
exercise intensities and types every 12-16 weeks to
keep your workouts enjoyable.

Of course, advance-schedule 4-6 workouts at the
beginning of the week.

YOUR BODY of EXERCISE

Habit #5   Balance your BODY of EXERCISE

A BODY of EXERCISE includes cardio, strength, flexibility training, and relaxation. Balance is achieved by representing all four disciplines of exercise to the degree that each addresses your specific needs and goals.

Modify your BODY of EXERCISE as your needs, desires, and goals evolve. The sample workout schedules I outlined in Habit #4 exemplify a balanced Body of Exercise.

Explore the benefits of each.

CARDIO

Upon rising in the morning, a typical pulse for a healthy woman is 65 to 70 beats per minute. Your heart rate doubles during cardiovascular exercise or aerobic training. Aerobic training is defined as having access to oxygen throughout the duration of your exercise.

During cardio or aerobic training keep your breathing pace between 65%-85% of your **maximum heart rate** for more than 20 continuous minutes.

I live in New York City. If I see my bus heading toward my stop, I charge down the sidewalk like a long-jumper to catch it. I have to. Everybody's in a hurry, even the bus driver. It's New York. I'm sure you've heard.

I'm usually hauling myself, my heavy boots, a purse, my gym bag, sneakers... My sprint is weighed down.

I have to run at full speed for 30 seconds to get there before the bus leaves. If you took my pulse, my heart would be beating at its maximum, so fast that I wouldn't be able to catch a deep breath or talk easily for at least 20 seconds.

Here's an equation to calculate a *heart rate maximum* :
220 – your current age. Let's use age 47. I was that age once.
The maximum heart rate = 173 beats per minute or bpm.

You could exert energy for your heart rate to rise to 173 bpm for 3 continuous minutes before you'd become uncomfortable. At that point, you'd need to slow your pace to catch a breath. **A heart rate higher than 85% of your heart heart rate maximum is your anaerobic threshold. A heart rate higher than 85% of your heart rate maximum is mainly for short bursts of exertion, strength, and power lasting up to 3 minutes, at which point it becomes hard to maintain.**

Remember, for aerobic training you need a sustainable supply of oxygen to your muscles and a breathing pace between 65%–85% of your *maximum heart rate* for longer than 20 continuous minutes.

Find the target aerobic heart rate using 220–age 47= 173.

Multiply .65 X 173. The answer: 65% of the maximum heart rate is 112 beats per minute or 112 bpm. Multiply .85 X 173. The answer: 85% of the maximum heart rate is 147 beats per minute or bpm.

Placing the first two fingers over the wrist pulse for one minute after aerobics, should equal a range between

112-147 beats per minute. Closer to 147 bpm is preferred.

When you CAMP OUT, you can plug your age into the equation to get your *maximum heart rate* and your *aerobic training heart rate*.

I've included another way to check your target heart rate intensity in the back of this book.

Try any of these aerobic exercises for 20-60 minutes ::

Aerobic dance class

Zumba

Kickboxing class

Aqua aerobics

Running/Jogging

Walking

Jump Rope

Step classes

Most dance classes

Skating/Ice skating/Rollerblading

Biking/Cycling (spinning is aerobic + anaerobic training)

Rebounding or jumping on a trampoline or BOSU

Regular, vigorous aerobic exercise near 85% of your heart rate maximum clears the plaque from your arteries. This helps prevent heart disease, the number one killer of women in the United States.

Highlighted Benefits of
Regular Cardiovascular Training

::

More stamina and endurance

Reduced risk of heart disease or stroke

Better circulation

Decreased blood pressure

Reduces bad cholesterol/Increases good cholesterol

Reduced stress, depression, and anxiety

Stronger immune system

Stronger bones from high-impact cardio

Increased range of motion

Increased coordination

Calmer mind

Improved sleep

Improved digestion

Reduced appetite

Burns calories

Cardio is necessary for a healthy heart, plus it burns calories and detoxifies your body. However, during the aerobic takeover in the 80s, women believed cardio was the main way to get lean. Please don't give cardio carte blanche if your goal is to lose fat and improve health. Muscle development is healthy, functional, and beautiful.

Dear woman,
Make muscle, not war.

STRENGTH TRAINING

Strength training is one of my favorite things to do. It changed the way I look and feel (and age). It's helped me handle the exertions of life. I am a determined, capable woman because of the tenacity and focus I've developed through weight-lifting.

Strength training is the practice of overloading your muscles using resistance from weights, bands, tubing, ropes, kettle-bells, bars, and your body weight. Strong, dense muscles increase your metabolism, strength, and stamina, improve your posture, increase bone density, and raise your overall level of confidence.

A body with muscle is gonna burn more calories than a body lacking muscle. And the obvious result of having muscle firmness is looking taut, sculpted, and shapely at every age.

LIFTING WEIGHTS WON'T MAKE YOU "DIESEL"
(UNLESS THAT'S WHAT YOU WANT)

For those who fear—*strong muscles equal BIG muscles*—be not deceived. It takes an overload of MASSIVELY heavy weight-lifting along with multiple supplements muscles grow to a massive size. Most women don't have enough natural occurring testosterone to develop large muscles. If you stay away from steroids, ladies, you won't need to worry about waking up one day with a tremendously thick bicep across your belly.

You will, however, get tight, strong, sculpted, and lean from strength training. Strength training can improve bone density, posture, and symmetric levels of strength. And if you practice strength training with proper form and alignment, you'll also develop the kind of body awareness you might not achieve from cardio. Clearly, you'll lose body-fat because muscle burns more energy or calories. You need muscle, especially because the average body gains 2% more fat every year after the age 35. After menopause, the lower body and abdominal areas tend to gain fat. Strength training will combat these issues.

Highlighted Benefits of
Regular Strength Training

::

Increased power, endurance, and strength

Increased circulation

More lean muscle, shape, and tone

Faster metabolism

Higher calorie burn

Lower body fat percentage

Stronger bones

Improved posture

Improved body awareness

Improved self-confidence

Improved balance

Decreased stress, depression, and anxiety

Calmer mind

FLEXIBILITY TRAINING AND RELAXATION

These two modes of exercise are often discarded as viable for fat-loss and health. However, for sustained fat-loss, both are necessary.

Cynthia and Amber attended 6:30 am spin classes on Tuesdays, Wednesdays, and Fridays before work. After three months, Cynthia dropped 22 lbs and Amber lost 17 lbs. They credited their spin teacher, Darnel, for changing their bodies.

While both ladies typically arrived for class early to secure a bike, they'd leave five minutes before the class was officially over. They'd skip the stretching portion.

It took a few weeks before Darnel questioned the ladies. They said they needed extra time to shower. Darnel expressed the importance of stretching major muscle groups after each workout. Tight leg muscles could potentially cause injuries to the knees, hips, and back. Cynthia and Amber promised they'd stretch in the shower.

Three weeks later, Cynthia came to class alone. When Darnel inquired about Amber, Cynthia shook her head. "Oh, it's bad. Amber has had pain and swelling in her knee for a few weeks. She's going to rehab now. Her physical therapist told her to lay off the bike for a while. I don't know what she's gonna do to keep her weight down, Darnel."

Cynthia stretched with the class from that day onward.

Stretching after your workout, when your body is warm and pliable, helps prevent injuries. Stretching speeds muscle recovery and lessens muscle pain.

Stretching increases the range of motion. There is a deliberate connection between the potential for strength and an increased range of motion. Imagine a high kick with a tight hamstring, the muscle on the back of your leg. The height of the kick is limited by the resistance of the tight hamstring. The pelvis would need to tuck under to help lift the tight leg. The force from tucking the pelvis combined the velocity of the kick could injure the lower back or strain the hamstring. A stretched hamstring releases the kick with less resistance.

Muscle tightness impedes circulation. This could cause headaches, neck aches, muscle strains, and prolonged muscle soreness. A decreased range of motion from tight muscles usually results in structural imbalances that, potentially, change the shape of your body. Can you take the shape of slumped shoulders and a forward extended neck? This position can lead to respiratory and circulation problems, headaches, back, hip, and knee pain. And it increases your risk of stumbling/falling.

For a structured stretching and balance practice, attend a yoga, Pilates, or Melt Method (foam roller) class. Otherwise, stretch for 5–15 minutes minimum after every workout. Stretch quadriceps or front thighs, hamstrings or rear thighs, your back, gluteus maximus also called glutes, and your triceps after every workout.

Highlighted Benefits of
Regular Flexibility Training

::

Increased range of motion
Increased circulation
Improved posture and alignment
Improved body awareness
Reduced risk of injury

Reduced muscle soreness

Reduced joint pain

RELAXATION TRAINING

Eastern healing modalities like yoga, Tai Chi, and Qigong have continually promoted the health and energetic benefits of conscious relaxation.

BECOME WATER

Relaxation and meditation is like Water to the Fire of cardio, strength training, and some styles of yoga and Pilates. Water types of practices are relaxing and restorative for the mind and body. Fire activities are expressed through physical exertion using force and power, vigorous breathing, and resistance. Your body needs both Fire and Water activities.

When you practice a relaxation technique that involves deep, focused breathing, you benefit from the happy endorphins, same as you would experience during a Fire activity. However, during the Fire activities your arteries constrict, your pulse is elevated, digestion is halted, and your muscles are generally tense. When you practice relaxation or a Water type of activity, your heart rate slows. Muscular tension subsides. Digestion improves allowing for easy elimination through urination and defecation. The nervous system can relax and rejuvenate.

Imagine what might happen if your body solely practiced Fire activities without Water. Excessive stress and tension of mind and body.

Imagine a body mostly engaged in Water type practices without Fire. Slower muscular alertness and reaction. Reduced speed, power, and force.

Put the Fire out with Water. Consider Water types of practices when you advance-schedule your Body of Exercise. Stretch your major muscles and relax your mind with a few minutes of deep breathing or a lovetruth practice after your workouts. And add a form of meditation.

MEDITATION INCREASES YOUR ENERGY

You can relax in a Yin style or Restorative Yoga class, Tai Chi or Qigong class, or practice some form of a meditation. Meditation will make you aware of the tension in your body and your mind so you can release it. The deep breathing helps discharge mental and physical stress by altering your biochemistry. Meditation reboots your energy for clarity and decisiveness.

Meditation might feel boring at first. You'll crave it after you feel the benefits.

Try any of these forms of relaxation/meditation:
1. Listen to music or affirmations with up-lifting messages while soaking in an Epsom salt and oil-essence bath.
2. Stroll through the park while you observe and listen to nature.
3. Improvise a dance with your eyes open or closed
4. Read a spiritual text that focuses on possibility, connection, appreciation, or love.
5. Swing or rock in a chair or hammock
6. Practice yoga nidra [a full-body relaxation and meditation typically following asana practice in traditional yoga].
7. Sit. Engage deep breathing. Do this before and after you VISUALIZE your lovetruths and during stretching time.
8. Journal your feelings and goals.

9. Do light housework silence or sit in silence.

Relax in meditation for 5-30 minutes at least <u>two times a week.</u> Engage in some form of relaxation practice every day for at least 5 minutes.

Highlighted Benefits of
Regular Relaxation or Meditation

::

Regulated blood pressure

Decreased stress, depression, and anxiety

Decreased muscle tension

Improved immunity

Calmer mind

More clarity

Improved sleep

Increased concentration

Increased intuition

Improved digestion and elimination

Reduced joint pain

Reduced appetite

Balance your Body of Exercise based on your BODY TYPE

There are 3 somatotypes or general body shapes.

Ectomorph.

Think of a naturally lean-looking body with generally low body-fat deposits. These types tend to lose weight quickly. Examples: Carrie Underwood, Gwyneth Paltrow, Cameron Diaz, and Sarah Jessica Parker

Mesomorph.

Imagine the naturally muscular-looking body. Remember the girl in high school who looked like she worked out all the time, though she didn't (ever)? Mesomorphs have low body-fat deposits and show muscle easily.
Examples: P!NK, Angela Basset, and Holly Hunter

Endomorph.

Think of a body with rounded shoulders and thick thighs. They carry more body-fat than the other body types. Examples: Queen Latifah, Alicia Keys, Adele, Serena Williams, and Marilyn Monroe

The celebrities mentioned are fit examples of these body structures.

TRAINING FOR FAT-LOSS

Ectomorphs are notably thin. Though they're perceived as *naturally* skinny, they may still carry excess belly-fat relative to their frame. **To reduce fat, they benefit from short, intense cardio sessions (20-30 minutes) 2-3 times a week, with an emphasis on building muscle with strength training, Pilates, and/or yoga 3-5 times a week.**

Why? Too much cardio or long cardio sessions will burn away their muscle. Ectomorphs need to strengthen their heart and lungs with aerobic training but greatly benefit from increasing muscle for bone density, stress reduction, and to reduce belly-fat.

Ectomorphs can increase strength and muscle definition with 8-10 reps per set. They can lengthen their rep pace with practice time-under-tension training. Time-under-tension is slow-rep training. Spend several seconds on the positive and negative portions of each rep. Imagine 4 counts to lower your push-up and 4 counts to push back up. Or 4-counts to curl your bicep, 4-counts for the negative. Each rep is slower than just one count down, one count up.

Ectomorphs can also use explosive strength training and plyometrics like jumping squats, jumping push ups, and hitting a boxing bag. Explosive strength training is recommended for mesomorphs, also.

Mesomorphs show muscle definition easily. They generally have less body fat than the other somatotypes. **For fat-loss they benefit from short, intense, heart-strengthening cardio sessions (30-45 minutes) 3 times a week and strength training 2-3 times a week.**

Because mesomorphs can look more muscular than other somatotypes, they can add an additional 30-minute cardio session each week to alter their aesthetics and reduce muscular thickness and definition.

Similar to ectomorphs, mesomorphs can burn away their muscle if they overtrain with excessive cardio sessions.

Mesomorphs are natural body types for fitness and bodybuilding competitions. For mesomorphs who want to increase muscle definition but not increase muscle size, focus on increasing the reps of body-weight exercises. Yoga and Pilates are recommended for this and every somatotype.

Endomorphs tend to have more difficulty losing body fat. They benefit from adding both short, intense cardio workouts and long, moderate-intensity cardio sessions (45-75 minutes) 4-5 times a week. Strength training is suggested 3-4 times a week. Use weights, bands, tubes, bells, or body-weight. Endomorphs can focus on lifting weights in the 12-20 rep range. **Endomorphs benefit from 5-6 total days of exercise per week to reach their fat-loss goals.**

Your body could be a mix of somatotypes like ecto-meso and meso-endo, but obviously not ecto-endo, as they are complete opposites. I am a meso-endo combo. You can determine your Body of Exercise by considering your somatotype or somatotype blend. Remember every body type needs to advance-schedule time for flexibility and relaxation for recovery.

Don't be fooled by covers. Even though ectomorphs look thin and mesomorphs look fit, they may still experience chronic stress and elevated blood sugar levels. Also, a substantial accumulation of body-fat around the abdominal organs could signal a health issue. Every BODY benefits from the medicine that a full Body of Exercise provides.

Some research discredits the existence of somatotypes. But if you happen to be an endomorph who knows it's super hard for you to lose weight while you watch your muscular, mesomorph friend look fit after two weeks of focused exercise, you know there's some validity to somatotypes. Use these guidelines to start your workout program.

CHECK-IN

Balance weekly workouts with a Body of Exercise that addresses your goals, body type, and fitness level. I moderately tweak the workouts I give my clients by juggling the types of exercises, the pace of the reps, shortening the rests between exercises, etc. Small changes to a workout program can increase muscular strength, stamina, and flexibility.

Everybody needs to advance-schedule time for flexibility and relaxation training.

The workout suggestions for the somatotypes are generalized. After you've consistently exercised 4-6 days a week for more than four months, you'll better understand how to arrange the Body of Exercise modalities to meet your goals.

After four consistent months of training, assess and modify your Body of Exercise. Tweak the type, duration, intensity, and frequency of your workouts. Re-assess your workouts every 6-9 months thereafter to meet your changing needs and goals.

CAMP OUT

PRACTICE THE HABIT

Habit #5 Balance your BODY of EXERCISE

Which somatotype or somatotype blend best describes
your body type?

Make a list of the kinds of exercises and relaxation
techniques you like best.

Advance-schedule your Body of Exercise every week.
You can mix cardio, strength-training, flexibility, and
relaxation/meditation into a single workout.

Sunday

Monday

Tuesday

Wednesday

Thursday

Friday

Saturday

Equation to calculate your aerobic heart rate zone for your cardio session:

220

-age

This is your MAXIMUM HEART RATE (This rate is difficult to maintain for more than 3 minutes.)

Your targeted aerobic heart rate range is between 65%-85% of your MAXIMUM HEART RATE.
Aim for 85% of your MAXIMUM HEART RATE.
X .85 = this is Your Aerobic Heart Rate goal in beats per minute or bpm.

Each of the 8 habits of *The RiTual* must be practiced if you want to lose fat and improve your health. Singling out your favorite two or three habits might work initially, but you want long-term success.

I mention this because we're about to look at how food contributes to fat loss. Some folks skip the exercise and mind-set stuff and focus solely on food. Some sign their **weight-loss will** over to ~~a DIET~~ a restrictive eating program that doesn't factor regular exercise. Some folks wanna shed weight without the sweating. Diet-only weight-loss isn't a form of holistic health. It might not be sustainable, either. A fat-loss program should transform your body and mind. Spooning yourself around a fat-loss program that features a nut, a fruit, and a special energy bar won't be transformative. You are a body, a mind, and emotions. You are the result of your behaviors, beliefs, and dreams. Consider your whole self in your health practice for sustainable results.

DON'T INSULATE. REJUVENATE.

What you eat matters. It accounts for 75% of your fat-loss success, which is why people grope at diet programs. Working out 4 days a week does not give you a pass to eat whatever you please. You won't enjoy a banging body if you eat foods that insulate instead of rejuvenate you. To become lean, healthy, and happy, you need to know which foods give you energy and longevity and which foods lead to undesired heaviness and coma-like lethargy.

Food is your medicine and your fuel. Food provides nutrients. It supports your muscles. It impacts your digestion. It can improve your sleep. It can boost your mood. The type and the amount of food you eat matters.

I was overweight because I had a love/loathe
relationship with food. The smell and sight of it was my
siren song. I loathed that I didn't have control over how
much I ate. I would finish every morsel of food in view.
I really love to eat! I'd say to justify my behavior.
It was a lie.

Love feels good. When you love something, you
appreciate it. I shoved food between my teeth and barely
chewed. I didn't love food, I loved to *consume* it. I didn't
recognize food for any of its qualities beyond how much
of it there was for me to hoard and how fast I could
make it disappear. My bond with food was better
described as an addiction. I rushed food into my mouth
like it was a contest. I was never happy after eating.
I was ashamed. Being teased about it stoked my
addiction. I hid in my plate.

Back then no one knew how I felt, including me—till I
journaled. My journals revealed how hoarding food let
me bury my feelings. I wanted to openly display my Self
as a creative, artistic being and create a life to match. I
over-ate to suffocate my frustration about being referred
to as *weird and different.* Mindless eating packed me into
a fat suit that insulated me from revealing my full
expression of Self.

Can you relate?

What's your relationship with eating/food?

Write about it in your journal.

FOOD FREAKS FOLKS OUT

Eating either too much or very little food can become a way to hide. Food can reveal privilege and abundance or make you feel insufficient and disadvantaged. Giving, receiving, or even rejecting food can demonstrate love, respect, and control. The way you eat represents status, your emotional state, your beliefs, and your goals.

People freak out about food, especially when it comes to losing weight. The belief that food equals fatness is damaging and causes confusion.

Food is fabulous. It's your ultimate source of energy. In this next section you will learn why you can come to your plate with excitement, creativity, and real love for what food has to offer.

Habit #6

Fuel every 4 hours on workout days

Fuel every 5 hours on non-workout days

The type, amount, and frequency of the fuel
you eat is majorly important to your fat-loss results.

Fueling your body and mind with real foods made from nature, not laboratories and scientists, will make you lean and healthy. Eat real, natural foods. Does picking out the real, natural stuff seem perplexing? Hells yeah. I get it. This is not your fault.

You have been clobbered by ads that say burger-up and enlarge that carton of fries. Two fast tacos are more economical than a salad. The cheap, franken foods win more air-time. So, you buy the Whopper without the cheese and feed one of the buns to the ducks to be "good". Or you buy the frozen, already prepared 300-calorie boxed meals because microwavable anything is easier than 15 minutes of boiling.

When you select the so-called healthy groceries, you're misled by the kitten eyes on the labels that promise *wholesome* cereal, *fortified* white bread, *vitamin-infused* intelligent water. Meow.

EAT FROM THE GARDEN

Start with the first rule of healthy fueling: choose au natural. If it's grown in a garden or raised in the wild, choose it. Food that has been enhanced or somehow re-created should not make it into your cart. Foods with ingredients you can't pronounce unless you've had three years of college chemistry; skip that stuff. Check the back of the boxes, cartons, and canned stuff. Read the bottled, jarred, and bagged stuff too. Processed meats and meat from animals that have seen a needle are problematic.

Avoid "diet" foods. Anything stamped low-fat, zero fat, low-sugar, fortified, enriched, refined, milled, infused, low-calorie has probably got mysterious ingredients you can't pronounce, contain a secret sugar substitute, or are devoid of fiber. If the food has been "created" gluten-free but has a sorted list of lab ingredients, reduce the portion you eat. Brown rice, wild rice, oatmeal, and quinoa are naturally gluten-free. They don't need the kitten-eyed label. *Natural* is key.

Buy fuel in its most natural state as often as you can. Eat lean, grass-fed, wild, pasture-raised, whole, slow-cook, and 100% natural foods with low amounts of sugar.

WHAT'S RED, HOT, BUT SORE ALL OVER?

Inflammation.

It's 5 am and still dark outside. You're fumbling your way to the kitchen. As you approach the blender to make your morning protein shake, BANG! Your knee slams into the open cabinet door. (Don't worry. This'll never happen to you.) You survive a small wound that requires a bag of frozen peas and a band aid. The injured area turns red. It's tender and warm and slightly bruised. In minutes, it's a bump. You have a minor injury. Your body goes to work to heal it all the same.

Whenever your cells get banged or ruptured, they become inflamed. The soreness, swelling, and hot redness are physical barriers that rope off and protect you from bumping it again. It wants to heal in peace. HIP, if you will. This is what happens with acute inflammation.

Cellular inflammation is more serious, especially because it could last for months or years, as we've discussed before. If you experience *chronic* joint pain, high blood pressure, blood sugar issues, ulcers, irritable bowel issues like diarrhea or constipation, or persistent skin problems, your body could be expressing chronic cellular inflammation. **Chronic inflammation can be caused by consuming packaged, processed foods and eating a large volume of sugary foods.** Additionally, your cells become inflamed when you exclusively consume a high volume of acidic foods like processed cheese, fried foods, alcohol, sodas, beef, and coffee, **without balancing it by frequently consuming** alkaline foods including lemons, broccoli, avocado, coconut oil, sweet potato, and herbal teas. Chronic inflammation is a precursor to heart disease, allergies, depression, and cancer, if unaddressed.

I reiterate

This is not a diet book, food glossary, or cookbook.

We each have **individualized** and exact needs when it comes to the macronutrients: carbohydrates, protein, and essential fats. One plate does not fit all.

Please use the upcoming grocery charts of desirable and occasional macronutrients to *assist* in organizing your healthy eating plan. The foods on the grocery lists are the lean, nutrient-dense, natural, alkaline, primarily anti-inflammatory varieties suitable for the general population. These foods will provide your body with fuel, reduce inflammation, support fat-loss, and supply energy.

In short, an individualized food plan can be generated after reducing, eliminating, and adding certain foods, then recording the results. This process should take weeks, sometimes months. No general eating plan could figure your specific needs without an individualized trial and assessment as described.

Please consult a dietician or nutritionist for an assessment and a PERSONALIZED food plan that accounts for your specific body type, activity level, sugar sensitivity, and medical needs.

What follows are the optimum times to eat your fuel and suggested portion sizes. But first, I gotta put to bed the touchy, feely advice to *eat ONLY when you're hungry*. It sure sounds like a sweet conscious-minded approach. Good luck, though.

Eating when you're hungry is definitely the worst health and fitness advice ever. You will perhaps never meet a fitness professional with lean muscle, strength, and youthful energy who eats whenever they're hungry. They regularly practice fueling their muscles and body at specifically spaced intervals to support their energy, workouts, and evolving goals. Fitness professionals fuel to support their sleep schedules, they eat to stave off muscular atrophy (muscle loss), and to strengthen their immune systems.

On the contrary, before I became a fitness professional, I ate when I was hungry, which was constantly. I'd smell beef sizzling on the grill—SQUIRREL—I'd get hungry. I'd see icing-drenched cinnamon rolls at the mall—SQUIRREL—I was hungry. I'd starve for two days, get hungry on the third, and eat without stopping till the sixth.

Stress, anxiety, and depression can make you crave and devour sugar or salt, or choose to skip meals for days. A whimsical eating plan is not recommended for health.

If you wanna run a marathon, you don't go for a run when you feel like it. If you own a business, you don't make sales calls when you feel like making them. When you attend college, you don't study when you feel like it. If you want to be energized, you don't sleep when you're sleepy! If you do, there is no way you'll meet your goals.

When we get highly emotional or stressed we lack tummy clarity. We need to automate some decisions, Charlie Brown. The decisions that could get drowned in your emotional soup must be advance-scheduled based on your needs and goals.

What you eat and when you eat needs to become a **habitual,** otherwise each day's fluctuating thoughts and emotions could dictate how hungry you are. Your activity level and your health goals must dictate your eating plan if your intend to lose fat.

You are working out 4-6 times a week for at least 45 minutes. You need fuel to provide energy to your muscles. Food can't be any ole thing you grab at the

drive-thru because it smells cracklin' good. Food must
fortify you with the nutrients at intervals that'll support
your daily activities.

When I had my weight issues, my food-bully was that I
didn't know the difference between hunger and interest. I
rarely felt full after eating. When *food* became fuel, its
significance became apparent. I went from eating to hide,
to choosing fuel to charge my body with energy.

To tame my overeating tendency, I drew associations
with mental pictures to bring consciousness to my
choices. Looking at a cake-pan of overflowing macaroni
and cheese made my heart and belly swell as I
envisioned clogged arteries and indigestion. Skip.

A turkey leg and bright pompoms of broccoli at
Thanksgiving made my mouth water. I envisioned
ballerina-like collar bones, sculpted shoulders, and
ripped abs. It gave me a sense of excitement to eat
knowing I was feeding my health and vision instead of
my frustration. I automated eating to break the habit of
unconscious eating and over-eating.

See food as the fuel it is, and you'll be able to chew on
good vibes, confidence, and more nutrients.

HOW MUCH SHOULD I EAT?

A woman's total calories each day is determined by her specific height, weight, age, and body-type. Generally a woman between the ages of 30-50 who exercises 4-6 days a week needs 1600-2200 calories a day, more if she works out at athletic intensities. How in the world will you know if you're eating 2000 calories? Are you gonna count each calorie... every day... for the rest of your life? Seriously, probably not.

Are you willing to cook all your food at home where you can measure and weigh it? Okay, I did that once... three times, actually. I was training for my bodybuilding shows. For the shows you stand on stage with four small triangles (over your un-muscled parts) tied on with strings to reveal your muscled parts. You're judged by your symmetry and lean definition. No fat allowed. When clients ask if they can try the diet I used for bodybuilding, my answer is *No way! It's not sustainable!*

My bodybuilding diet was extremely rigid, time-consuming, and bland. Bodybuilding is a serious sport, an art form. Bodybuilders prepare in phases. The lifestyle requires that you schedule an *off-season* to give your body a rest from the intense training and restrictions.

A bodybuilder's eating plan is NOT SUSTAINABLE FOR
DAILY LIVING.

You can track your food every day without counting
calories. Let me shed light beams on the notion of
calories. They matter, and they don't matter. Food is
more than calories when it enters your body. When it
enters your body it becomes nutrition or fuel, or it
becomes stored.

A woman who wants to lose weight reduces her daily
calories from 1900 to 1500 a day. She eats 400 fewer
calories a day. Since one pound equals 3500 calories,
after 28 days she'll probably lose 3+ pounds.

That's 400 X 7 = 2800 fewer calories consumed per
week.
2800 X 4 weeks = 11,200 calories lost in a month.
11,200 ÷ 3500 = 3.2 pounds lost in a month.

However, if the 1500 calories she consumes include
orange juice, small pancakes, fruit roll ups, packaged
veggie burgers, boxed prepared meals, low-fat cookies
and sugar-free whipped cream, she will achieve a
"smaller" cream puff of a body. Just about all of those

calories come from sugar sources and processed foods. Her eating plan would be devoid of the nutrients she'd need to energize her muscles, workouts, and her brain.

Now, let's give her fuel. Pack her cupboards with slow-cook oatmeal and millet, flax and chia seeds, freshly blended almond butter, coconut oil, extra virgin olive oil, almonds, and avocados. Stock her fridge with grass-fed and wild caught meat and fish, pasture-raised eggs, home-prepared bean burgers, sweet potatoes, spinach and broccoli, pears, berries, and iced green tea. Eating fuel like this will help her body shuttle glucose into her muscles instead of her fat cells, charge her brain with energy, help her achieve deep sleep, and reduce cravings and boredom. She'll be tighter, leaner, and happier eating these foods.

Which body would you rather have?

To practice habit #6 of *The RiT* you won't have to pack miniature scales or calorie charts in your purse. Instead, pay attention to your portion sizes. Eyeball your macronutrient portions, carbohydrates, proteins, and healthy fats, and **eat with your hands.**

EAT WITH YOUR HANDS

For most meals EAT:

- a fiber-rich carb

- a lean protein

- a healthy fat

If you fuel every 4 hours, you will probably eat 3-4 times
per day.

For ONE or TWO of your main meals you can eat:

◆ a fist of protein

◆ one or two open hands of greens/veggies
(includes greens, colorful veggies)
and/or

◆ one palm (with thumb up) or 1/2 wine goblet of a
starchy, fiber-rich carb
and

◆ two to three fingers of a healthy fat

For ONE or TWO smaller meals or NUTRITIOUS BOOSTS
eat a full hand size portion of fuel that includes
a carb, a protein, and a fat
including the GREEN MUSTACHE

Read further to learn more about LEAN and GREEN meals, nutritious boosts, and green mustaches.

The **eat with your hand** portions loosely correlate to a quarter, half, and full cup measurement.

Overeating causes digestive issues, insulin resistance, inflammation, and pre-diabetes which is the gateway to Diabetes Type II. We'll look at the physiological problems of overeating in habit #7.

THE MAIN EVENTS

MACRONUTRIENTS

- *I'm on low-fat diet!*
- *I eat protein once a day.*
- *I really don't eat that many carbs.*

Do you trust your Carbs, Protein, or Fat to take care of your body? Who's the coolest macro between the three? Don't judge your macronutrients. They're good for you. Say it with me: *Macros are good for me—Macros are good for me.*

Okay, here's what you need to understand. Because no two bodies are exactly alike, you need to eat carbs, proteins, and fats to the amount that supports your individual body type AND activity level. Your carbs, proteins, and fats will continue to undergo assessment and tweaking as your body and energetic output changes. Macronutrient needs are a bit different for people over 50, but that's a discussion beyond this book. Uh-hum. If this is you (over 50 rocks), you could eat 2-3 meals per day and still feel energized. Listen, I'll write that book later. Eventually everyone will need it.

CARBOHYDRATES

I don't eat carbs. You don't need to eat carbs if you sit and stare at walls for 24 hours. You could starve yourself of carbs for weeks if you don't need to use your brain. In truth, your body might can survive for longer than you think without carbohydrates. But, you wouldn't be healthy without the nutrients from carbs.

If you exercise 4–6 days a week (and you are), your poor belly would squeak at alien decibels in hunger without carbohydrates. Your weak legs would spontaneously collapse without carbs. Ravenous, you might devour my shoe, the rotten banana peel in my gym bag, and the expired yogurt in the trunk of my car, if you skipped carbs for too long. In short, when you're working out using **The RiTual**, you need the energy, strength, recovery benefits, and brain food that carbohydrates provides.

Your muscles, liver, and brain rely on glucose delivered by carbohydrates. Without carbs, you forgo fiber, vitamins, and minerals. Skipping them for long periods could set your appetite to crave a binge.

Carbohydrate is not a bad word to a fit person. Carbohydrates include a wide range of foods. The high sugar varieties are responsible for giving carbs a bad reputation. They're the ones we tend to crave and overeat. Reducing or eliminating some of those carbs is a good idea.

Carbs have 4 calories per gram. You're not tallying calories with *The RiT,* but it helps to understand calories when you're making associations and configuring portions. You want to be able to identify the different types of carbs and become aware of the carbs that supply the nutrients that support your goals.

All carbohydrate calories are not created equal. Especially carbohydrates that are not created naturally. Carbohydrates include all starches like breads and pastas, potatoes, rice, beans, though some beans also have high amounts of protein, fruits and vegetables,. You can eat all the carbs mentioned as long as you understand **when** and **how much** will provide your body with fuel.

Consider the sugar-rich or starchy carbs. Say you habitually consume a large volume of starches and sugars (white rice, pasta, cereal, rolls, juices) or say you generally over-stuff yourself when eating any kind of food. High-sugar eating and overeating means insulin undergoes the exhaustive task of moving the excess glucose out of your blood and into your muscle, liver, and brain. If you over-eat or over-consume sugars regularly, you could develop *insulin resistance*. Insulin resistance is a petulant child, with crossed arms and a pouty-mouth, who won't finish dinner. "No more! No! I won't eat it!" That's what your muscle, liver, and brain cells say as they refuse to accept the excess glucose. There are cells that are happy to take your excess glucose, though—your fat cells!

All that extra glucose gets converted to fat. When this happens your body stops burning fat for energy because, well, there's so much extra glucose in your blood to use for energy, if needed. If the energy isn't needed, your simply gets fatter fat cells.

Most of the fat cells that take the glucose are located around your vital organs, the visceral fat near your abdominal area. These fat cells produce *cytokines*, inflammatory chemicals that cause other cells to become inflamed.

Exhale. Take a seat. You can keep this from happening.

RELAX, SUGAR

Carbs that contain high amounts of sugar ⟹ all breads including buns (wheat and the gluten-free versions), cereal, breakfast porridge, most pasta, white rice and white potatoes, tortillas and pitas, cornbread, biscuits, pancakes, muffins, doughnuts, cakes, cookies, crackers, pop tarts, sweetened drinks and juices, most desserts, ice cream and most yogurts, jelly and jam, honey, sauces and gravies, dried fruits, beer, and wine.

That's just naming a few. Excluding the white potatoes, white rice and a few others, most of these are carbs are not made naturally. They are made from ingredients that have been *processed, milled, refined, enriched, or engineered.* These are the sugars you want to reduce. Totally eliminate some of them. Replace some with a high-fiber carb.

A note about carbs labeled *diet*—skip these, too. *Diet* versions of these foods are not automatically a healthier option. When a *diet* version is created, you can bet it's been processed (code for adding unnatural ingredients), which could lead to issues in the gut and potential fat gain.

Diet versions don't get a pass. I used to think they did. Remember the Snackwell cookies from the 90s? If you don't, they were quarter-sized, low-calorie cookies. I'd eat a whole box by myself (about 90 cookies) while watching the Tonight Show with Joan Rivers. Did you just have a flashback? Me, too.

Instead of *diet* foods, choose small portions of whole, natural, high-fiber versions of starchy carbs/foods.

Here are a few carbohydrates made from nature. Sweet potatoes, quinoa, brown rice, slow-cook regular or steel-cut oatmeal, beans, all the leafy greens, carrots, root vegetables, cucumbers, celery, all onion and garlic varieties, broccoli and cauliflower, and all fruits and berries. Eat carbs that provide fiber, antioxidants, phytonutrients, and vitamins and minerals for fuel. Eat carbs that supply your muscles, liver, and brain with energy.

The RiTual without carbs sets you up for a binge. It's called THE CRAZINGS. You'll end up head first in vat of ketchup soup with fries.
Choose carbs intentionally.

EAT CARBS

Respect the **type** of carb and **portion size** and you'll lose fat. Choose greens and veggies like peppers, tomatoes, spinach, broccoli and cauliflower as your nutrient-dense, low calorie carbs. Eat them every day. Eat blackberries, raspberries, peaches, pears, and guavas.

Choose starchy carbs that are high in fiber. Choose sweet potatoes, slow-cook oatmeal, brown and wild rice, and quinoa. You're right. I haven't included pasta. Worry not. There's an Asian noodle, Shirataki noodles made from yam, that you can eat as a substitute. You won't miss the bloat from pasta. Shirataki noodles are translucent, slippery noodles that take on the flavor of your sauce and spices. They're naturally gluten-free, fat-free, and Kosher. I order the MIRACLE NOODLE brand from Amazon because they don't have fillers. It's the only brand I recommend. If you choose a different brand, read the label. Make sure the noodles only have 2-3 ingredients.

These yam noodles come in a clear bag of liquid. Rinse them well. Fill a pot with water to cover them and boil for 3-4 minutes. They have a smell that you may find off-putting (I don't). The smell goes away once the noodles are rinsed a few times, and you certainly can't taste the smell. I always wash the noodles—maybe you can taste the smell if they're not washed. I'll never know. Anyway, the fettuccine-cut noodles don't smell as much as the angel hair.

Eat your fiber-rich, starchy carbs 90 minutes before or after your workouts.
Avoid eating starchy carbs and fruits three hours before going to bed unless you have a workout scheduled in the evening.

BODY TYPE SPECIFICS

Ectomorphs tend to burn calories at a rapid pace. Based on **eat with your hands** recommendations, ectomorphs and mesomorphs may need to fuel with an extra portion of fibrous, starchy carbohydrates during one or two meals. Also, both ectomorphs and mesomorphs may benefit from eating 3-4 fruits a day.

I suggest that endomorphs fuel with an additional one-hand portion of vegetables during two of their meals to create fullness and extend the digestive process (the breakdown of fiber). The body actually burns calories during digestion. Fiber burns calories during digestion. Also, since endomorphs burn calories slower, eat no

more than 2-3 fruits per day and no more than a palm
of 2 starches daily.

GROCERY LIST OF
DESIRABLE CARBOHYDRATES

all green vegetables

all green leaves

peppers

tomatoes

zucchini/squash

cauliflower / broccoli

cabbage/ bok choy

all onions

garlic

chickpea pasta

Shirataki noodles

(translucent Asian noodles made from yam)

all fruits

berries, cherries, guavas,

pears, apples, peaches, plums,

oranges, grapefruits, all citrus,

pineapples, mangoes, papayas, melons, dates, figs,

tomatoes

slow-cook oatmeal

sweet potato/ yam

quinoa (also good source of protein)

chia seeds (also good source of protein)

brown rice

wild rice

beans (also good source of protein)

Ezekiel brand products

raw honey

(The starchy carbs and fruits are not desirable 3 hours
before bedtime, unless there's a workout.)

REDUCE the portion-size/ frequency or eliminate

root vegetables

all breads (except Ezekiel)

all pasta (except Ezekiel or Shirataki noodles)

white rice, white potato

yucca

soda, sugar, artificial sugar, fruit juices, pancakes, waffles,
muffins and doughnuts,
and the sweet C's—crackers, cookies, cakes, candies,
custards
and the other pastry-like treats, buns, and rolls
(reduce portion and/or frequency of wheat and gluten-free
carbs)

THE GREEN MUSTACHE

A NUTRITIOUS BOOST in a glass

I don't recommend a liquid diet of green mustaches all day, every day, though one green mustache every day is a recommended nutritious boost.

FRESH AND GREEN IS THE WAY TO DRINK CARBS

Drink greens once a day as often as 4-6 days a week. If you're not a vegan or vegetarian, it might slip your mind to advance-schedule vegetables. So, begin the habit of blending a 16-ounce (that's 2 cups) glass of nature's finest elixir.

Blenders save the whole food along with the fiber. Juicers press the fiber out. Use a super blender like the Vita-mIxer, NutriBullet, the NinjaKitchen System, or any blender that can grind at a speed between 600-900 watts. If your blender isn't powerful, try blending your ingredients in shifts. Start by blending the green leaves with a little liquid, then add the chunky items with a bit more liquid, and last add the softer ingredients plus protein, then blend.

The green mustache substitutes as one of your daily meals or your nutritious boost (explained later). I like to drink my greens within an hour following my workout or as the last meal of my day. If I drink my greens at night, I reduce the fruit to half of what I'd use during the day to cut sugars. Any time of day is a good time for a glass of nutrients and anti-inflammatory health.

Here's a delicious green mustache recipe.
1 palm of fresh or frozen spinach or kale
1 organic celery stem
or
8 sprigs of parsley
quarter-size chunk of peeled ginger
one banana
half an avocado
handful of nutritious or more
1 cup of water to your taste
BLEND till greens are fine or in small bits.
Serves 2
Cut the recipe in half to serve one person.

Drink fresh! Chewy the leaf bits to release enzymes that aid digestion.

Ginger root is spicy. I blend a large chunk into my green
mustaches. Spicy makes me smile. Experiment with
ginger till you know what suits your palate. I have clients
with an avocado phobia. Green mush isn't appetizing to
some. I can't think about green mush too long either, so
let me get to the point. When you blend avocado into a
protein shake or green nutritious boost, it loses the
avocado taste and texture. Instead, it turns the beverage
into ice cream-esque deliciousness. The avocado and
banana together make your drink taste more like a
dessert than a nutritious meal.

For protein and extra nutrients, add two scoops of **vanilla
whey, pea, or vegetable protein powder (20-25 grams) or
a teaspoon of chia seeds, nutritional yeast, kelp powder,
bee pollen, and sea moss powder to your green
mustache.**

Lick your green mustache lip with satisfaction.

PROTEIN

Protein has 4 calories per gram. Again, you're not under
the minutiae of counting calories but comparing
macronutrients when you eat with your hands.

Protein doesn't create muscle. It heals muscle. During strength training your muscles undergo microscopic tears. Your body uses protein to repair the muscle, making it stronger and more developed. Protein allows you to reap the reward from your workout. Muscle can improve your posture, strengthen your bones, and help you burn more calories each day.

It's a 95 degree beach day. You and your bestie, Gloria, are chatting on your towels. You've been attending 2 strength training classes and 2 boxing classes every week for 7 months, and it's noticeable. When Gloria sprays your back with SPF, she comments on your muscle tone. Gloria's right. Your shoulders are sculpted. Last summer you wore a one-piece because you didn't feel confident .Now your mid-section looks like it did in your twenties.
You both weigh the same. Gloria attends a cardio session three times a week. She's lost a few pounds, but her body doesn't show any muscle tone under her cover-up.

You recline into your beach chair to read from your Kindle. Gloria checks her phone. **Because you have more muscle, you're burning more calories than Gloria as you both sit absorbing beach air.**

Protein is the building block for muscles, hair, cartilage, bones, nails, and blood. You need protein to make enzymes and hormones. Eating protein with carbohydrates can manage blood sugar elevation. Protein eaten with vegetables digests well.

Like carbs, the amount of protein **you** need is specific to your bodyweight and the type, frequency, and intensity of your workouts.

The recommended amount of protein (RDA) is 0.8 grams per kilogram of bodyweight. That looks like this quick conversion for a 170 pound woman:
170 lbs divided by 2.2 kg.
170 lbs = 77.1 kg
77.1 kg X .8 = 61.7 grams a day.

The Recommended Dietary Allowance does not consider one's daily activities or volume of intense exertion. In other words, this recommendation is good for someone who moves very little each day. Sedentary individuals do not need extra protein.

Fuel your body based on your activity level and body type. When practicing *The RiT* your general protein prescription is: eat protein grams equal to 40% – 50%

of your total weight. This will support your activity level using *The RiT*.

So, if you weigh 170 lbs, eat between 68 – 85 grams of protein each day. This amount of protein will also make up for eating fewer calories from starchy carbohydrates and fruits.

Athletes increase their protein. I eat roughly 60% of my total weight in protein grams. My bodyweight is 149–152 lbs. (Most women have a weight range of 2-3 pounds that fluctuates daily.) Since my strength training workouts are heavy and intense, I consume 70–90 grams of protein each day. When I competed in bodybuilding I consumed up to 140 grams every day. During my bodybuilding training, my weight dropped from 162 to a competing weight of 140 pounds. I worked out 6 days a week, with 2 workouts daily. Closer to competition, I ate 120–140 grams of protein while reducing the other macronutrients. I drank protein shakes twice a day in addition to eating four small meals to meet my physical demand.

Once again, I do not recommend my bodybuilding protocol, because it's not sustainable. Neither are most diets, which I also do not recommend. Stick with eating

40% - 50% of your bodyweight in protein grams. Keep in mind, you are consuming protein based on your activity level, exercising 4-6 days a week, and your body weight. If your conditions change, you'll need to adjust the amount of protein grams up or down accordingly. It always goes that you should consult a professional dietician/nutritionist who understands how to fuel your personal exercise and fitness needs.

GROCERY LIST OF

DESIRABLE PROTEINS

lean, organic poultry/pork

lean, organic, grass-fed or wild meat

wild-caught or small fish

shellfish

fermented tofu

tuna or pink salmon (canned + fresh)

cottage cheese

tempeh

organic milk

nut milk

greek yogurt with cultures

beans, lentils, chickpeas rinsed / soaked

pasture raised eggs

whey or vegetable protein powder

chia seeds (also a source of carbs)

quinoa (also a source of carbs)

nutritional yeast

<u>REDUCE or Eliminate</u>

fried protein, packaged and boxed protein (the kinds with several ingredients like packaged foods), most deli meats, most cheeses, hormone + antibiotic-injected proteins

Here's a glance at protein grams and portions for some foods.

1 large free-range egg = 7 g

3 oz. of wild salmon = 19 g

3 oz. of grass-fed beef = 21 g

1 can of tuna in water = 40 g

1 cup of 2% milk = 3 g

1 cup of almond milk = 1 g

1 serving of 2% Vanilla FAGE greek yogurt = 12–19g

1/2 cup of cooked lentils = 9 g

1 scoop of Gold Standard Whey protein powder= 24 g

1 scoop of NOW Foods pea protein powder = 24 g

1 scoop of Orgain Vegetable protein = 21 g

Carbs, proteins, and fats have been at the center of a forty-year battle to see which is making us fat. Research currently clears all three of their bad reputations. Each of them deserves a place on your plate. Sugars, GMOs, trans-fats, artificial foods, and medicated proteins are the culprits killing our efforts to get lean and stay healthy.

EAT FAT

As your fat therapist, I need you to understand why essential fat makes you healthy and happy. For years you've been told to go low-fat, no-fat, ghost-fat, and hide from fat. Once you understand how healthy fat contributes to your personal fitness, health, and beauty goals (yes, beauty goals), you'll certainly find space for it on your plate.

At 9 calories per gram, fat has twice as many calories as the other macronutrients, hence the reason it was feared when we thought fat was evil. But nature-made fats have desirable body and beauty functions. Essential fats keep your skin and eyes from becoming dry. Essential fats keep your hair from getting brittle. Fat lubricates your joints. Fat protects your nerves. Fat reduces depression. Fat is needed to absorb vitamins A, D, E, K. Fat is necessary to regulate the female reproductive system.

Visualize fat foods. What do you see? Slices of pizza hanging from trees by their cheesy strings? A drum-line of fried chicken parading at half time? If so, divert your inner-vision to a scene in paradise. You're on a remote island. Four birds serenade you from the palm tree. A ripe coconut falls, landing softly on the sand. Perfect timing, because you were standing under that tree two minutes ago. There are plump avocados in the garden ready for picking. You'll dine on them at sunset along with the lightly, coconut-oil sautéed sardines you caught during morning fishing. Healthy fat abounds.

Mend your relationship with this f-word.

In the current American diet, we consume too many omega 6 fats and under-eat the more desirable omega 3 fats. Omega 6 fats consist of vegetable and corn oils, sunflower, soybean, and cottonseed oils, mayonnaise, cookies, and cakes.

Omega 3 fats, the preferable fats, are found in walnuts, flax seeds, chia seeds, brussel sprouts, watercress, seaweed, and several fishes: wild caught salmon, lake trout, mackerel, herring, fresh tuna, anchovies, sardines, and oysters.

Americans ate a 1:1 ratio of omega 6 to omega 3 fats before the fast food saturation. Now we consume omega 6 fats to omega 3 at 16:1. The research suggests lowing the ratio to 5:1 or 3:1 omega 6 to omega 3 fats. Modify omega 6 fats by changing the type of oil you use for cooking. Organic coconut oil, walnut oil, and extra virgin olive oil are healthy sources.

Your fuel list of healthy fats is shorter than the other macronutrients. The portion sizes are smaller, also. Be mindful not to over-eat the fats on your grocery list beyond the recommended **eat with your hands** portions. This is especially important with nuts! Because nuts come in large containers, divvy out the three-finger portion (10-15 pieces) into Ziplocs or small dishes so you won't be tempted to munch 'em like popcorn.

FAT THERAPY

Fat will give a feeling of fullness so you won't over-eat protein or carbs. Remember, essential fats make you gorgeous and slowdown aging. Your knees will thank you.

GROCERY LIST OF

Healthy FATS

avocado

coconut oil

extra virgin olive oil

grass-fed butter

nuts and seeds & naturally blended nut or seed butters

fatty fish: sardines, salmon, herring, cod, Atlantic mackerel, lake trout

You don't see fried foods on this list, do ya?
Try your best to eliminate them.

Reduce or eliminate these, too.

packaged and processed foods

margarine - which is a processed food

ALL fast foods,

ice cream, desserts, gravies and sauces

[Also refer to the foods listed earlier
to increase your Omega 3 and decrease Omega 6 foods.]

A NATURAL HAPPY MEAL

Add natural extra flavor to your meals, and start a party
on your tongue and in your cells.

HERBS

Basil and oregano are superstar herbs. You've probably
eaten them within the last week. Try other natural flavors
from your garden. Pick rosemary, parsley, dill,
peppermint, cilantro (and coriander seeds), sage,
tarragon, and thyme.

Herbs de Provence is one of my favorite herb
concoctions. It's a blend of herbs that grow in South
France including summer savory, rosemary, thyme, basil,
tarragon, oregano, and lavender. Check a brand for dried
lavender. It's not always included. Lavender elevates the
flavor of this blend.

SPICES

Push table salt away. It's heavily processed. Switch to Himalayan Pink Salt. It's pure salt, rich in iodine.

If you're used to adding lots of salt to meals, substitute a spice instead. There are many anti-inflammatory benefits in turmeric, cayenne, and ginger. Turmeric is a cancer preventative. There's a compound in cayenne that's widely used in over-the-counter arthritis and muscle-pain creams. Consider adding cinnamon, cloves, nutmeg, mustard seeds, and black peppercorns from a pepper grinder to your meals. I sprinkle cinnamon into my filter when I brew coffee. The spices add sophisticated flavors to your dishes. You won't miss the salt.

Snack might as well be a four-letter word.

Re-think the word "snack".
I tell my clients to eat a small meal during the day for an energetic boost, to prevent a blood sugar crash, and to stave off the possibility of bingeing during the next meal.

I avoid calling these small meals snacks. Snack might as well be a four-letter word.

SNACK evokes memories of childhood foods that weren't necessarily healthy. Remember the kindergarten days of juice boxes and graham crackers? Teachers served six colorful M&Ms on a red napkin, fruit cups with peel-off lids and finger-length spoons, Nilla Wafers on a brown paper towel—sugary treats. Aka snacks! Remember snack-time when grannie gave you processed applesauce, an orange popsicle? Yep, it makes me smile, too, but the *snack* habit.... Your PROGRAM might have formed an unhealthy association to that *SNACK* word.

Grown-ups eat midnight sugary snacks and visit snack machines for more sugar. A candy bar, a bag of corn chips, a big bowl of popcorn, 6 servings of "healthy chips", a meal replacement bar loaded with fructose corn syrup— Did someone say sugar or or did you say snack? This is getting confusing.

That's why you can scratch the word ~~snack~~ and replace it with **nutritious boost**. Choose food that provides nutrition, balances blood sugars, and reduces stress.

Pick a **nutritious boost.**

These qualify as nutritious boosts:

1. a palm of almonds and one banana
2. one handful of cherry tomatoes (drizzle olive oil and add basil slivers) and one boiled egg
3. one handful of blueberries or blackberries or raspberries with 10 walnuts
4. 2 handfuls of edamame
5. one halved boiled egg with mustard, cayenne, pepper, and pinch of pink salt with a pear
6. a handful of turkey jerky and an apple
7. 2% or whole Fage yogurt with added berries, chia seeds, and/or a teaspoon of raw honey
8. one slice of Ezekiel bread/toast with almond butter
9. one peeled and sliced cucumber marinated in vinegar with cayenne, pepper, and pinch of pink salt
10. a green mustache! Blend a palm of two to three greens—spinach, parsley, celery, cucumber, or kale plus a sweet food; either half a beet, a carrot or a fruit halved or whole (apple, pear, berries, banana) with water and ice. [you can add protein powder, ginger, spices, flax or chia seeds, half an avocado as you choose] Drink 12–16 oz fresh!

(Eat a variety of GREENS. Too much spinach—though it's
hard to eat too much spinach—can cause kidney stones.)

WHEN SHOULD I FUEL?

Fuel your body every 4 hours.

Here's a sample fuel timeline:

Wake at 5:30 am

Meal 1 Morning meal 6:00 am

Workout at 7:30 am

Meal 2 Nutritious boost at 9:00 am

Meal 3 Afternoon meal at 1:00 pm

Meal 4 Evening meal LEAN and GREEN at 5:30 pm

Bed at 9:30 pm

Here's another fuel timeline featuring an evening workout.

Wake at 7:00 am

Meal 1 Egg meal 7:30 am

Meal 2 Afternoon meal at noon

Meal 3 Nutritious Boost at 4:30 pm

Workout 6:00 pm

Meal 4 Evening meal 8:00 pm

Bed at 11 pm

On the two or three days during the week when you don't workout, extend time between meals.

On non-workout days you can fuel every 5-6 hours. Like this.
Wake at 6:00 am
Meal 1 Morning meal or protein shake at 6:30 am
Meal 2 Afternoon meal at 12:00 pm
Meal 3 Nutritious Boost or GREEN MUSTACHE at 5 pm
Meal 4 LEAN and GREEN meal at 7:30 pm
Bed at 11:00 pm

You <u>can</u> eat in the evening. When you practice *The RiT*, make your last meal jolly, green, and nutritious. **Make it a LEAN and GREEN meal and eat it 3 or more hours before bedtime.**

Three reasons why you can eat in the evening:

1. Eating three hours before bed gives you time to digest your meal. Your sleep cycles won't be interrupted, and you'll experience deep, restful sleep.

2. Eating a healthy lean and green meal as your last meal of the day minimizes fat storage and creates satiety

through the night. Wild caught salmon, lean chicken thighs, or an omelette for protein. Broccoli, spinach, arugula, watercress, and romaine salad. Add a drizzle of extra virgin olive oil (an essential fat) and balsamic vinegar with herbs and spices to flavor.

3. If you workout in the evening, **you'll need nutrition for your muscles.** Here's the happy rub: **After an intense evening workout you can add a fibrous starch and/or a healthy fat to your last meal.** Eat protein to slow the absorption of sugar (carb) and to aid in muscle recovery. Stay lean and green, but add a small palm-sized portion of brown rice, wild rice, sweet potato, Ezekiel pasta, or one slice of Ezekiel bread and/or a healthy fat like a quarter section of avocado/two tablespoons of guacamole, a palm of almonds, walnuts, or pumpkin seeds, one tablespoon of nut butter, or a teaspoon of coconut oil, to list a few healthy suggestions. Adding a small portion of healthy fat after your workout will help regulate your blood sugar and aid with restful sleep.

EMOTIONAL SOUP

During the beginning of your fitness program you may notice you don't have an appetite after your workouts. Amped with enthusiasm, you might feel inclined to skip meals, convincing yourself it's okay because you usually eat too much anyway.

Early enthusiasm neutralizes after a month or two on a fitness program. Within weeks you might notice you feel hungrier because you're lifting weights and exercising longer with cardio. This roller coaster of feelings and eating patterns can shake up your program from structured and advance-scheduled to random and emotionally driven.

Starving weight off usually ends in binge city (binge city stays open all week and you don't need a reservation). Structure your workouts and fuel by advance-scheduling them from the beginning. Remain consistent. Even as enthusiasm ebbs and flows, do not eat when you feel like it. Eat for fuel every 4 hours on workout days. Eat every 5-6 hours on non-workout days. Follow *The RiT*.

Go for nutrients. Eat au natural foods that elevate your energy, support your workouts, repair and build muscle, balance your blood sugar, and enhance your mood.

Advance-schedule your healthy eating plan at least 6 days of the week, every week. Advance-schedule and pre-select your nutritious boosts.

Advance-schedule the days you plan to have a cheat meal.

Wait. I've gotten ahead of myself. That's the next habit.

Each week, you get to cheat.

CHECK-IN

Eat to rejuvenate, not insulate.

Eat to fuel your mind and body.

The best food on earth is from the earth. The other food-stuff, food made on an assembly line, is probably responsible for expanding your fat cells.

Healthy "wild" eating is more tasty than boxed macaroni and sliced wiener casserole. Raise your thumb if you agree.

Choose a nutritious boost, not a snack.

Habit #6 Fuel every 4 hours on workout days (every 5 hours on non-workout days)

Review your grocery lists of desirable macronutrients. Which foods are you going to buy for sure?

Advance-schedule your fuel and nutritious boosts after you read the next habit.

LEAN HAPPY HEALTHY YOU Journal

Do you have a tendency to overeat?

How does your body feel when you overeat?

How do you feel when you overeat?

Why do you think you do it?

Does food comfort you? Which foods?

How does your body feel after you eat them?

List 5 unhealthy foods you eat regularly?

List 11 healthy foods that you eat regularly.

How do you feel about eating healthy foods?

List a few ideas of how you can add flavor to meals
with spices and herbs.

What have you learned about food?

What have you learned about your eating habits?

What happens when you smell a pan of freshly baked chocolate chip cookies and there's no one around?

Habit #7   Eat one CHEAT meal each week.

After you've been practicing *The RiT* for five consecutive months, you can eat a *cheat* meal 2 times per week.

HANDLING THE CRAZINGS

Diets suck the marrow from your soul. They do. What usually happens when you can't stomach the diet any longer?

Deprivation usually unleashes a feeding frenzy. Without warning, the hunger monster embodies you and your commitment. You need a healthy eating plan that extends beyond your January pinky-promise and beyond the weekend retreat of juice cleansing.

Our bodies are in constant fluctuation ladies. Blame this on hormones, and you wouldn't be wrong. If your environment, internal and external, was steady and predictable, I'd say stick to an exclusive program of eating wild, healthy foods every minute of every hour. *Never cheat*, I'd say. But if you never got another chance to lick hot wing sauce from your fingers, we might find you insane and three feet deep in the Chinese buffet one day.

You gotta handle those *crazings*, I mean, cravings.

Sometimes crazings are triggered by childhood memories. The smell of baking brownies reminds you of rainy Saturdays playing CONNECT FOUR in the kitchen. Earth, Wind, and Fire jams remind you of Milk Dud and Orange Crush breaks at the roller skating rink. Those are my memories from Iowa. How about your memories?

A healthy eating plan can aid in 75% of your fat-loss and mental health success, and you must take that seriously. Still, I don't want you to step on the tail of your hunger monster.

Instead of waiting for everyone to go to bed so you can inhale four pieces of Aunt Carole's carrot cake, go ahead and eat a small slice at dinner. Eat that thing you crave.

Eat a slice the size of your palm and enjoy it—but only once a week.

When the corners of your lips purse and you're teetering on insanity because you've committed to eating only healthy food for the rest of your life, you might as well have dropped your iPhone in a public toilet or given your Pit Bull your 1970s Chanel handbag to play with. It's okay to have a cheat meal.

All cake is not lost when you want to be healthy. Once a week feed The Crazing.

Indulge in a small portion of something you're salivating for, but only **the size of one hand-portion with the thumb up.** (Hey, looks like you can have that pasta after all.)

It's called *cheating.* I encourage it. Cap those crazings, or they'll storm you. Quell the urge, erase an option for guilt, get your cheat behind you, and then get back to feeling sound about your quality decision to live healthy.

During your first 2 weeks practicing *The RiT*, Do NOT CHEAT. Strictly advance-schedule and log your fuel from the grocery lists of desirable foods.

During your third week, eat one cheat meal per week. And after you've practiced **The RiTual** for five consecutive months, you can eat up to 2 cheat meals per week.

Fitness professionals have been eating cheat meals for years. As of late, there's been a new conversation about whether folks should avoid *cheating* altogether. The argument equates cheat meals to letting alcoholics have one drink a week. First of all, you *have* to eat. No one has to have alcohol. And although food addiction is a significant pathology, the other 7 habits of **The RiTual**, especially the habits of mind and heart, are scaffolded to support you so cheat meals won't take you from your resolve.

Cheat. Semantics matter to me, as *SNACK* became **nutritious boost**. A *cheat* meal is meant to be a cheat! No hiding the intention. A cheat meal is a built-in gasp of air. It's a blip off the path of restriction. *Cheating* frees you from diet prison.

The cheat meal gives you autonomy. Like being able to wear paisley printed socks with your school uniform, you get to choose ANYTHING, of the recommended portion size, to eat as your cheat. You'll become adamant about what to choose for your cheat meal. You won't waste it on any ole thing.

My cheat item is typically a gooey chocolate brownie. It's the one I dream about on long bus rides, the one that melts in my mouth and sticks to my teeth. It feels sensual to my taste buds, guilt-free decadence, heavenly bliss. I will only eat a brownie if it fits a certain criteria: moist, glistening, memorable after the first bite. I never waste my *cheat* on an ordinary brownie.

Because I've been diligently advance-scheduling my *cheat* meals, I don't respond to OPOs and OPAs persuading me to cheat all the time. Before practicing **The RiT,** I'd sample large tastings whenever asked by OPOs and OPAs to try a dish. Now, I show discretion. I will eat one to two *cheats* per week. A dessert or meal item I consider a *cheat* must look, smell, and taste exactly as I desire or I won't eat it. If I taste a *cheat* and don't like it, I won't finish it. I will not waste a *cheat* opportunity on an item I don't want. This has contributed to mindful eating. It will do the same for you.

Why *cheat?* You'll think about food differently.

1. After choosing healthy, natural foods for 2-3 months, your taste-buds will dull the desire to scarf down some of the foods from your past PROGRAM. You'll naturally want to cheat less often, perhaps once a week, or you'll naturally cheat with smaller portions.

2. When you eat a smaller cheat portion, your PROGRAM wires a new relationship to the cheat item. Your confidence skyrockets when you gain this kind of self-control.

3. After engaging in 4-6 workouts every week (and looking fine and fit because of it), you will no longer make a pact with disappointment by inhaling a box of powdered mini-doughnuts during a successful workout week. You'll become more aware of how your workouts, fuel, and cheats are sustaining your results.

Why *cheat?* It helps you lose weight. Your body benefits by eating a calorie-dense food cheat food once or twice a week.

1. Leptin, a hormone made primarily in your fat cells, regulates your appetite and signals cues of fullness

your brain. Leptin decreases after 72 hours on a low-calorie diet plan. The *cheat* meal usually increases your caloric intake, which helps reset your leptin gauge. It's important to know, over-eating and bingeing upsets leptin, the signal that tells you to stop eating. Leptin resistance is a precursor to insulin resistance, Diabetes Type II, and obesity.

2. Ghrelin, produced by the stomach and pancreas, signals to your brain that blood sugar is low. It stimulates hunger. When you restrict calories for long periods, ghrelin kicks into high gear, potentially increasing hunger, thereby causing the dreaded binge.

3. Once you've practiced **The RiT** consistently for more than nine months, your digestion won't easily accept some of the old unhealthy foods you used to eat. The physical discomfort from trying to digest those processed, fatty, greasy, over-sweetened foods will temper your desire to crave them. One hand-sized portion with the thumb up of your cheat food will be the portion you'll want because you'll be used to digesting this smaller size.

Strictly advance-schedule and log your fuel from the Grocery Lists of Desirable Foods ONLY for the first 2 weeks practicing *The RiT*. This is referred to as CLEAN EATING. Exclusively eat healthy foods. Consider it a "soft" cleanse as it will detoxify the body and reset your taste buds.

During the third week, eat 1 cheat meal per week during your first five months practicing **The RiT**. Eat up to 2 cheat meals each week after you've been practicing **The RiT** for five consecutive months. **Each cheat meal is the size of one hand with the thumb up.**
Eat a cheat meal. Don't have a cheat day.

The best time to plan this indulgent hand-size with a thumb up meal is during a day when you're planning a strength training workout or a high-intensity cardio workout.

My *cheat* meal options include:
1. Six pieces of sweet, sticky, and very, very spicy chicken wings.
2. Three slices of super thin crust pepperoni pizza
3. A gooey brownie, but you knew that—and it's smaller than a hand portion, but all I need, uh—I mean all *you* need is one.

4. Three scoops of Ben and Jerry's chocolate chip cookie dough frozen yogurt (I'm not an affiliate for the company. I simply love their frozen yogurt.)

Isn't is exciting to know you can cheat once or twice a week? Make sure your other meals come from real, nature-made foods in the suggested portion sizes, all advance-scheduled.

Obliging my *cheat* is how I bypass the urge to binge. I don't have to arm-wrestle any crazings after my *cheat.* I calmly get back to the business of eating for fuel. The world goes back to spinning, the clocks go back to ticking, I go back to fitness. But, when I don't oblige my *cheat*, my crazing grows a head, tail, and fangs. The crazing attacks me when no one's around to witness the streaks of fudge smeared up my cheeks.

CHEAT MEAL RULES OF CONDUCT

Buy your cheats on a per-cheat basis!

1. Don't grocery shop cheat foods in advance. Keep cheat foods and other temptations out of your cabinets, car, locker, pocket, purse, and pocket.

2. Buy cheat foods on a per-cheat basis (the day you're gonna eat them).

3. Don't buy the stuff you are going to eat during cheat meals in quantities larger than the amount you're cheating with, and don't buy them till you're gonna cheat with them (I'm repeating that for a reason).

4. No matter how controversial to the rules of etiquette, do not volunteer to doggie bag the un-eaten or extra desserts or fried foods from a dinner party or holiday get-together to eat later as your cheat. **Just say no.** Don't take temptation home with you.

5. If you eat your cheat at someone's house, you don't have to finish it if it's larger than a hand with a thumb-up. No matter what anyone tells you, no one ends the starvation in impoverished areas by eating your large servings of toxic foods in America. There are better ways to end the food crisis in the world. Eat less.

Please check here (www.feedingamerica.org) for more information.

CHECK IN

Don't let the stuff that tempts you into *the crazings* rent space in your kitchen or they'll gobble up your might.

Buy your cheat when you are ready to eat it.

To cleanse your palate and your body, EAT CLEAN from the desirable grocery list during the first 2 weeks practicing **The RiT**.

Thereafter, eat 1 cheat meal per week for five months practicing **The RiT** and up to 2 *cheat* meals per week after you've been consistently practicing **The RiT** for more than five consecutive months. Remember, each cheat meal is the size of one hand in portion with the thumb up.

CAMP OUT

Habit # 6 + # 7 Advance-schedule your fuel and cheat meals every week

1. Use a fuel [food] journal or use your LEAN HAPPY HEALTHY YOU journal. Advance-schedule (pre-plan and log) the foods, times, and portions for each of your meals and cheats for both workout and non-workout days.

2. Log for 6 months. After 6 months of advance-scheduling you will be conscious of the food that loves your body. Return to keeping a fuel log if you find it difficult to regulate your eating plan for fat-loss.

LEAN HAPPY HEALTHY YOU Journal

Make a list of the options you'll eat for your nutritious boosts.

Make a list of foods that qualify as *cheat* meals.

What scares you most about having *cheat* meals during the week?

What scares you about EATING CLEAN for two weeks?

How would you feel about strictly EATING CLEAN with NO *cheat* meals at all?

After you EAT CLEAN for two weeks, write about how you feel.

After 9 months, ***The RiT*** will become your lifestyle.

At this time, I recommend a reboot or cleanse.
Cut cheat meals and EAT CLEAN for 2 weeks like when you started The RiT.

Reboot every 4 months thereafter **or** for the first 2 weeks of every season. During the 2-week cleanses, eat strictly from the Desirable Grocery List with an emphasis on vegetables, fruits, eggs, fish, and healthy fats.

MEET YOUR MAKER

This habit is a part of Habit # 6, but it's so important it needs its own section.

WATER: DRINK at least half your body weight in ounces of WATER per day.

DRINK more water on intense workout days and hot days.

Would you enjoy pain-free knees or would it be okay to feel like there are rocks in your knees when you stand up to leave?

Would you like to digest your food and absorb the nutrients into your cells? Do you want to flush toxins and waste regularly from your body or would you rather be deficient of vitamins, sluggish, and constipated?

Do you want to have soft, supple, clear skin or do you want dry, cracked cheeks that suggest you're 10 years older than you are?

Do you want to lose fat? Or would it be okay to grow an inch more fat on your back each year?

WATER is for you if you desire better digestion, clear skin, and pain-free joints. If you don't care about these results, consume copious amounts of bottled fruit juice, soda pop, and alcohol instead of water.

IS BOTTLED JUICE UNHEALTHY?

Ban bottled juices from your existence. Bottled juices are addictive and often consumed in large portions. It mainlines straight to your fat cells when you drink too much of it. Perhaps you choose bottled juice to score vitamins. Did you know that vitamin potency dissipates when juice is exposed to air and light? Juice in clear bottles that have been shipped and stored for weeks is colorful liquid sugar by the time you take a sip. Bottled juice is like a snack containing enough calories to equal a small, sweet meal. When you drink bottled juice with a big meal, it spikes your blood sugar level. If this pairing becomes a habit, insulin resistance will be looking to add you as a friend.

If you're a bottled juice-aholic, slowly wean yourself off the weight-gainer. Mix 2 parts water with 1 part of your bottled juice to equal a total of 16 oz. After a few weeks, you'll be able to turn away from bottled juice altogether.

Juice is not sinful. Drink real juice, made from live, squeezable fruits, served in a 12 oz container. Or better, as learned in habit #6, combine one fruit with a bouquet of green plants and give yourself a fresh green mustache most days of the week. To modify sugar content, blend your juice with one sweet ingredient like a banana, a carrot, a beet, or half two fruits. Add veggies like celery, cucumbers, kale, spinach, and/or parsley, and always drink your juice blend fresh.

MERGE

Meet your maker. Your body is more than 70% water. Water is you. Merge. Drink water.

If you've been opposed to drinking water, you simply must get over it. Or drink plain seltzer.

Elevate your water or plain seltzer by adding a slice or two of cucumber with the skin on. Thoroughly wash the skins to remove pesticides. Cucumbers help repair electrolyte imbalances by providing potassium. They're high in Vitamin K which helps build strong bones. Munch the slices when you finish your water.

You can add a sprig of mint or an orange slices, grapefruit, lime, ginger or a lemon slice to your water.

Begin your day with a glass of hot or cold water. Add a squeeze of lemon to improve digestion, add potassium, alleviate joint pain and inflammation, and to strengthen your immune system.

There are amazing benefits from nature's liquid.

Benefits of
Drinking Water

::

Hydrates your cells
Helps you digest and absorb food better
Enhances circulation
Moves nutrients to your organs
Helps to remove toxins out of your body
Keeps your joints lubricated
Helps metabolize fat

That's a heap of reasons to rock your boat in the water.

Drink at least 50% of your bodyweight in water ounces.
I drink approximately 100 ounces of water daily, which is way more than half my bodyweight in ounces. When I'm

at home, I drink water from a gorgeous goblet. Goblets beautify everything, appreciating my water into an elegant beverage. I also serve my morning oatmeal and my cheat pasta portions in a glass goblet.

Drink your water in a fancy glass. If you're out roaming, invest in a BPA-free water bottle. Bisphenol A or BPA is what makes plastic containers toxic. The plastic leaches into your water whenever the plastic gets warm. Think about the great water warehouses around the country storing millions of plastic water bottles with toxic water awaiting thirsty stores and lips. I shed a tear for those non-biodegradable plastic bottles strewn across the land and ocean.

LIFE FACTORY makes reusable, BPA-free glass water bottles. CamelBak and Nalgene make reusable, BPA-free plastic water bottles. Buy some beautiful goblets for regal water at home. Maybe keep your glass or metal goblets in the freezer if you want a cold, frosted cup of nature's gift.

The tap is my main source for water. If you choose tap water, let it run for 15-30 seconds before you fill your container. Stagnant water runs through the pipe, the fresh stuff flows afterward. To know whether your tap water is pure, google your government's water standards or check with the Environment Protection Agency. If you prefer a water purifier on your tap, google Consumer Report's reviews on water purifiers. Aquinas 3-stage Under the Counter and WaterChef got good reviews in 2016. You can also use a pitcher with a disposable filter like Clear2O Water Filtration Pitcher, plus Brita and Pur get good reviews. Check out glass or PBA-free plastic pitchers.

HEALTHY BEVERAGE OPTIONS

Coconut Water

Read the label to make sure it's 100% natural coconut water with no additives. Coconut water will be the **only** ingredient listed. Nature made this drink, so don't buy substitutes made in a factory. It costs companies significantly less to give you a little bit of coconut water and fill the rest with their addictive flavor enhancers. Be choosy. Read the label.

Real 100% coconut water has potassium and sodium and a natural sweetness. The best time to drink 12-16 ounces of coconut water is after an intense workout session. The sugars will directly replenish the glycogen used from your muscles.

Though coconut water is a great beverage and a healthy choice, don't drink it all day and definitely skip it at bedtime. It's not calorie-free like water. One-coco-a-day is enough. Drink it before or after your workout or in the morning.

Some believe you acquire a taste for coconut water. Isn't that the case with most new things? This will definitely be the case if you're used to drinking sodas, diet sodas, and heavily sweetened bottled juices. You'll have to wean your buds from the alluring sweetness from the aspartame used in sodas. Aspartame, also called Nutrasweet, hasn't been proven harmful to most healthy people if it's consumed in small doses. However, studies show that those who frequently nosh on foods and drinks containing aspartame may have an altered sweet-tooth tolerance. Perhaps heavy aspartame connoisseurs think fruits don't taste sweet and vegetables taste like compressed paper. According to the research, those who consume aspartame tend toward having weight issues as they may crave foods that are higher in sugar. Solution: skip the fake sugar.

Tea

Green tea has abundant antioxidants that reduce free radicals in the body. Free radicals damage skin cells. Free radicals can contribute to heart disease and cancer. When you slice an apple in half and expose the flesh to air it turns brown. This is similar to the way free radicals affect your cells.However, a squeeze of lemon juice on exposed apple flesh keeps it from browning. Green tea is like a squeeze of lemon to your cells.

Some studies have proven that green tea reduces LDL cholesterol levels, balances blood sugars, and aids in digestion. Substitute green tea, iced or hot, in place of artificially sweetened beverages and high-sugar juices to reduce the intake of sugar calories.

Choose green tea, oolong tea, or herbal tea. They all get two thumbs-up. Try adding natural flavoring instead of sugar. Steep your tea with ginger slices, cinnamon sticks, mint leaves, star anise, and/or citrus fruit slices. If you must have sweetness, use half a teaspoon of local honey.

PARCHED AND PUCKERED OUT

A cramp in your ab during SOUL CYCLE. Going to bed with a low-grade headache after Bikram Yoga. Groggy and tired after your morning run. These could be signs of dehydration. Sure they could also be signs that you're a SOUL CYCLE beast, that your Bikram teacher had a grating voice, or that you were up all night because your neighbor played ABBA for 6 hours. Most likely you need to drink more water, half your body weight in water ounces. Drink more when it's hot and if you sweat more.

Bad breath and alligator skin are signs you've been dehydrated. Don't let it come to that.

CHECK IN

255

Perhaps you tend to grab coffee or tea. Don't forget to gulp water.

There is plenty of water in fruits and vegetables, too. Fueling your bod with a fruit and several vegetable servings per day, including your GREEN MUSTACHE, helps to fulfill some of your water needs.

Hit Trader Joes with your checklist: 100% coconut water, green and herbal teas, and a BPA-free water bottle.

Drink your water from the crystal goblet you bought for special occasions.

CAMP OUT

PRACTICE THE HABIT

Habit #8 DRINK at least half your BODY weight in ounces of WATER each day.
DRINK more on intense workout days.

How much water will you drink per week?
Your bodyweight ÷ 2 = # of ounces per day

Do you have a vessel that can measure your water ounces? For example, use a 6 oz. goblet or a 32 oz water bottle.

Do you have a BPA-free water bottle?

Think through your day. When is a good time for a water break or ten?

NOT OVER TILL THE FIT LADY ZZZZs

Habit #8 Sleep 6-9 hours 6 nights a week.

7-8 hours are optimal.

Aim to go to bed at the same time and wake at the same time most days of the week.

I used to be proud of myself for functioning with 4 hours of sleep. Functioning with little sleep ages you, weakens your immune system, and makes it harder to lose fat. Sleeping is a panacea for good mental and physical wellness.

DEEP REST helps you lose fat.

When I took my iPad in for service last July the attendant ran some diagnostics then asked if I ever turned it off. Well... no. Should I? I mean, it's an Apple product. Are we supposed to turn Macs off?

She explained that although Macs are superpowers, they need to shutdown periodically so the system can reboot. Your body, similar to my iPad, needs to be turned off so it can reboot, update, and run all the programs you've put in it. Your body needs to rest.

**Quiet your mind and body at the end of each day.
You need to rest.**

Sleep on average 6-9 hours per night. Research suggests 7-8 hours is ideal to rejuvenate healthy adults. Book-end your day. Go to bed at the same time and wake at the same time most days of the week, with a buffer of 60 minutes at either end. For example, go to sleep between 9:30 pm-10:30 pm, wake up between 5:30 am-6:30 am. This helps to condition your body to a sleep rhythm. Creating a sleep rhythm will help remedy problems falling asleep or struggles to get out of bed in the morning.

SLEEP IS THE PANACEA

Sleep helps to keep the fat away. According to the research, the metabolism is slower in adults who sleep fewer than 5 hours per night and is optimal in those who sleep at least 6 hours. Both **protein** and adequate **rest** repair and regenerate muscles with strength and hypertrophy. Quality sleep contributes to three aspects of your health and fitness: it helps your muscles repair and grow stronger by awakening the hormones that heal the bodily tissues, it decreases a peptide that causes hunger and cravings, and it puts the hormones that cause stress to bed.

Leptin is a hormone that tells the metabolism to either operate efficiently and burn fat, or slow down and hold onto fat. It also sends a message to your brain that you've had enough to eat. The peptide, ghrelin, tells your stomach—*Grrrr, keep on eating.*

Without deep, regular sleep, your leptin decreases (ugh... slower metabolism and a body that holds onto fat) and ghrelin increases (eek...! Increased hunger and cravings). Missing out on deep zzzzs makes you ravenous during the day and, sometimes, during the night! I've had clients infected by poor sleep. They've confessed to eating full meals in the middle of the night.

Typically, your cortisol levels should drop at bedtime. If your mind knocks round the details of life, you won't be able to slumber because cortisol levels are spiked.

Elevated cortisol can cause cravings. High cortisol levels at bedtime might inspire you to visit the fridge or the "vineyard". If you reach for a glass of Merlot or a cold Heineken Light to calm your nerves before bed, you're causing more stress and fat. The alcohol enters your body as **sugar** causing fat storage. Alcohol also disrupts your sleep cycles, in particular your restorative REM and deep sleep, both necessary for fat-loss and mental health.

Deep sleep produces HGH [human growth hormone]. HGH helps metabolize fats and synthesize proteins for muscle repair and strength. HGH also increases kidney flow and filtration, enhances the immune system, and increases collagen synthesis and cartilage growth. Your natural production of HGH decreases as you age, but regular exercise and 7-9 hours of regular sleep re-stimulates its production. Isn't that good news?

I'm not saying you'll be healed and happy enough in 6-9 hours of sleep that you can skip your doctor visit. But it helps! Setting bedtime and waking time at the same times each day is a natural panacea for your mental and physical wellness and strength.

One-third of your life is spent sleeping. Sleeping is no waste of time.

To create an environment for restful sleep, try one or each of these suggestions:

1. Make sure your bedroom is dark. This is the most important part of your bedtime ritual.

Researchers have noted that with the invention of electricity came more cases of depression, mental health issues, and weight-gain issues. Internet addiction has ramped these issues up. Light interferes with your natural bio-rhythms. Your mind needs to know it's nighttime. Turn the lights down one hour before bed. Read (preferably not horror or anything by Nostradamus). Skip the 24 hour news. Take your thumb off scroll and tuck your phone away. In fact, hide your phone in the kitchen drawer. The light on the screen and the alerts keep your mind stimulated.

2. Play soft music or a soundtrack from nature Alexa.

But make sure you cover the screen. The glowing light will keep you awake. Computer lights inhibit the melatonin needed to dim your internal lights and quiet your mind.

3. Eat your last meal 3 hours before bed.

A heavy meal before bed stimulates digestion. You might feel uncomfortable, crampy, or need to use the toilet when you're in bed. Your organs need to relax to help you fall asleep.

Make your last meal of the day a lean and green one. If you become ravenous at bedtime, which may happen if you've had a couple intense exercise days back to back, add an essential fat to your meal like a fist-size portion of salmon, or a quarter of avocado, no more than 8 almonds, or a tablespoon of naturally ground almond butter to keep your blood sugar stable overnight.

4. Take a warm bath with Epsom salts.

Dry your body after the bath in a dimly lit room and slather cool lotion over your skin. Lavender and frankincense essential oils in the water or lotions soothe and calm your nerves. End your bath with a cup of herbal tea infused with a cinnamon stick, mint leaves, or lemon.

Epsom salt is Magnesium Sulfate. It helps flush toxins from your body, reducing inflammation. It also increases serotonin to help you relax. You'll absorb the magnesium sulfate through your skin while you soak in the tub.

Use 1/2 cup or less in a full warm tub of water. I soak three nights a week in Epsom salts. Too much Epsom salt could cause health problems for some, including constipation because of the magnesium—certainly not what you're looking to experience. If you don't have time for a bath, soak your feet in Epsom salts.

Make sure your essential oils are pure and high quality. Consult a professional when choosing essential oils and using Epsom salts. Epsom salts and essential oils are not recommended if you're pregnant or have sensitive skin.

Are you rolling your eyes wondering how the h*^l you'll be able to arrange a spa-style ritual before bed every night? Every suggestion here will reduce stress and set you up for better sleep. They are worth implementing. Schedule them as you've advance-scheduled your workouts.

For example, if you decide that Sundays, Mondays, and Thursdays are the days you most need to de-stress, mark your calendar ad tell everyone in your home you're booking the bathtub for an 8 o'clock salt soak on those nights.

Prep your environment for your nighttime ritual.

Advance-schedule time today or tomorrow to select a book, appropriate music, buy greens at the Farmer's Market or get frozen broccoli at BJ's, and/or get Epsom salts at the dollar store.

Pre-select your outfit for the morning, CHARLIE BROWN; pack your gym bag, and prepare your fuel and nutritious boosts for the next day.

Your bedtime habits will soon become automated and you won't be able to imagine how you've ever slept without them.

Sleep 6-9 regulated hours at least 6 days during the week. This prescription is general. For example, I've trained older adults who thrive with only 6 hours of sleep per night with a 10-minute nap on some days. Ten years ago I regularly slept 8-9 hours most nights. Now that I go to bed at 11:00 pm and wake at 5:30 am, I feel rejuvenated after 6 1/2 hours. Plus, I plug in a 10-minute nap two days a week on my intense workouts days. If your lifestyle is such that 6 hours of sleep is actually a luxury, thank heaven for the NAP.

SIESTA

Naps belong to the energetic toddler. Naps are coveted by basement dwelling twenty-somethings who haven't realized there's a world outside Facebook.

Your cat loves the nap. Your pup wants a nap. It's customary in many countries to pause for siesta, a town-wide nap. Why did you stop taking them in the first place?

The nap is an opportunity to neutralize stress. The nap reboots and refreshes your nervous system. The nap is especially for you if you exercise 6 days a week. You need the blip of rest to regulate your blood pressure and repair your muscle. The nap is for you if your mind works on overdrive.

A 10-15 minute nap is great, so get one. However, if sleeping in the back of your classroom while your middle school students take their Science exam could get you fired, Ms. Jackson, there's another way to take a rest.

A 5-minute meditative break, called a *mental massage*, provides the same benefit or better as the nap.

**Close your eyes and focus on your breath. Let breath
massage you from the inside out.**

THE MENTAL MASSAGE

Sit in a private place like a bathroom or the back of your
classroom during your lunch break. For 5 minutes, close
your eyes and take a few slow breaths. Imagine your
face and shoulders relaxing. Scan your body for tension.
We hold tension and stress in the neck, shoulders,
eyebrow and mouth areas, hands, and low back. With
slow, deep inhalations, direct your breath to these areas.
Feel tension leave as you release the breath in slow
exhalations. Don't think about the future or the past. Let
your breath massage your body. Feel the breath as if
you can see it.
You will feel calmer.

I begin my mental massage by thinking LET ME BE
KINDNESS or I CHERISH THIS CLARITY or MAY MY
WORDS INSPIRE. I proceed with my deep breathing
body-scan. I end by silently repeating my chosen
intention. After, I go back to work.

If you can't find a quiet space for mental massage, you
can still practice. The space must only be private in the

sense that no one can disturb you. Sit in your parked car at the grocery store. Sit for a mental massage at the bus stop, as long as there's no one asking you how to get to Broadway and 82nd street. You can practice the mental massage anywhere for 5 minutes of rest.

Add one or all of these practices to your bedtime ritual:

- Practice a calming Yoga sequence followed by a 5-minute mental massage.

- Write in a gratitude journal and visualize your lovetruths.

- Say a prayer of gratitude and empowerment.

CHECK IN

We spend two-thirds of life sleeping. Getting 6-9 hours of regular sleep regulates your metabolism, reduces cravings, and neutralizes stress. Sleep provides a portal for dreaming, where you process your emotions.

Go to sleep at approximately the same time and wake-up at close to the same time each day. It creates a sleep rhythm so you can fall into sleep and awaken naturally.

Take a 10-minute nap once or twice a week, especially if you are exercising intensely or not getting adequate sleep at night.

Spend 5-30 minutes in a mental massage. The mental massage provides space for conscious breathing and mental rest.

CAMP OUT

Habit # 8   Sleep 6-9 hours every night.

Go to sleep and wake up at approximately

the same times most days of the week

What time will you go to bed and wake-up most days of
the week?

What is your new bedtime ritual?

What do you need to prepare for your bedtime ritual?
Epsom salts? Essential oils? A yoga practice? A playlist
of nature sounds?

When might you be able to advance-schedule one to
three naps per week? For how long?

LEAN HAPPY HEALTHY YOU Journal

What are your obstacles around practicing a nighttime

ritual?

How might you overcome them?

Write about your experiences implementing a nighttime

ritual.

Can you advance-schedule 1-3 mental massages

per week?

What is your intention?

Write about your experiences using the mental

massage and intention.

The RiTual

1 Set meaningful goals

2 Practice lovetruths

3 Advance-schedule your workouts and your fuel

4 Workout 4-6 times a week for 45-90 minutes

5 Practice a balanced Body of Exercise

6 Fuel every 4-5 hours and drink water

7 Cheat one to two times a week

8 Sleep 6-9 hours each night

Did it take you two weeks to get to this point in the book? I hope so, because that means you've really been engaged, taking notes, and starting to implement *The RiT.* Even if you read slower, you're here now. This is exactly where you need to be.

As I've said before, I've worked with lots of minds and bodies. I've heard everything, every obstacle, every concern—everything. Obstacles from the OPOs and OPAs are prevalent. But obstacles also arise from your own internal voice.

You will being facing personal concerns as you up-level your health. Focus on implementing the tools and habits to remain faithful to your meaningful feelings and vision.

During PART FOUR, I'll highlight the obstacles you might face. If these are your challenges, I'll make a few suggestions to help you handle them.

PART FOUR

TRUST

BACK AWAY FROM THE SCALE

The bathroom scale seems the obvious tool to measure your progress, right? Not necessarily. Back away from the scale. It won't always tell the truth.

Smash the scale. Is your forehead's crinkled? Okay, let me put it this way. If you have one, you don't need to drop it off the balcony. But swear to me you'll only use it three or four times a year.

Your scale might not validate your progress. It could misguide, and possibly, depress you more than reveal the forward progress you're making toward your vision.

Because you are practicing the 8 habits of *The RiT* every week, you *will* lose body fat. And you *will* gain dense muscle that reshapes your body, strengthens your bones, and increases your metabolism. These positive these results *can't* be represented by the scale.

Worse case scenario ➥ The scale dials down during weeks 2 and 3. The dial fails to move during weeks 4 and 5. Then the dial goes up during week 6 and stops again on week 7. You'll try re-calibrating the scale. Maybe you'll shake it, kick it, take it into a different room

—anything to make it work the way you want. Panting to gain composure, you assume—*muscle weighs more than fat.*

Nope. It doesn't. One pound of muscle weighs one pound, and one pound of fat weighs one pound. Yet, fat and muscle do not look or feel the same, nor do they treat your body the same way.

A pound of muscle takes up far less space than a pound of fat, making your body appear smaller and tighter. Read that sentence again. Let's say a pound of fat looks like a shoebox of pink cotton candy and a pound muscle looks like a filet mignon—sorry vegetarians. Imagine the size difference.

If after two months with **The RiT**, you're able to lose eight pounds of fat and gain five pounds of muscle. The scale says you've lost three pounds. Only three pounds lost? Your reaction might warrant a scale kick. Just three pounds of weight loss might send you to the cupcake shop for a box of six. Just three pounds lost after eight weeks of uninterrupted hard work and dedication is potentially so disappointing that you might take a hiatus from advance-scheduling your weekly workouts or give up on your vision altogether.

Be advised, your efforts have been physically and healthfully noted. You've toned up, up, and away from the eight pounds of gooey fat. Remember, that fat weight is gone. You've reduced your risk of heart disease and Diabetes Type II. You've strengthened your bones. Your digestion and elimination have improved. You're probably now or soon will be wearing a smaller dress size.

Shame on that scale for misrepresenting you! If you solely depend on the scale, you'll weep when you should shake your booty and give high fives.

So when should you weigh yourself and when should you back away?

Weigh yourself three to four times a year. Schedule your first weigh-in as soon as you begin *The RiT* so you can establish a baseline. Then weigh yourself at the beginning of week 4 and week 9. Weigh-in again at the beginning of week 16. After that, **weigh-in once every four months to 6 months.**

Unfortunately, having a scale in your bathroom is like having a bag of Oreos in your purse. I've known a client to wake-up, pee, brush her teeth, and weigh herself. Then she'll go to gym, tie her sneakers, fill her water bottle, and weigh herself again. I'm not finished. She'll do a cardio kickboxing class, steam and sauna, and weigh herself again. And this is all in the same day. Every day. Once we instill habits, they get stored in our PROGRAM and feel like the normal thing to do. Do not make weighing yourself all the time a habit. If that locker room scale winks at you, look away.

Here's the exception—If you have more than 30 pounds or up to three dress sizes to lose, use the scale <u>once every two weeks for three months</u>, then follow the schedule I mentioned earlier in *The RiT.* Your results will be dramatic in the beginning, then they'll taper off.

If you have 10 pounds or less to lose, the results on the scale will probably deceive you. When you have fewer pounds to lose, weight-loss is slower. I'll explain more in the MAKE PEACE WITH TIME section.

MEASURE YOUR PROGRESS

If you don't have skin-fold calipers that measure body fat or the means to weigh yourself underwater, use these four methods to track fat-loss and improved health.

- Use a tape measure.

- Look at your body: take a picture and check the mirror.
- Use your clothes. Your zipper won't lie.
- Let your annual doctor's report measure your success.

Your weight would be a greater issue if Zuckerburg forced you to add it to your Facebook url ➠ facebook.com/**152pounds**. Contrary to what we fear most about scale weight, nobody gives a hoot what you weigh. Only you and your doctors need to know that number anyway.

▪ Measure the circumference of four essential body sites.

A tape measure costs a buck at the dollar store. Invest.
☑ Measure your dominant arm halfway between the shoulder and elbow
☑ Measure your waist an inch below your belly-button
☑ Measure your dominant leg halfway between the knee and hip
☑ Measure your hips around the widest part of your buttocks.
Chart these measurements when you begin practicing *The RiT*, then again at the end of weeks 4, 9, and 16.

Measure your body sites every four to six months thereafter.

DATE	Arm	Waist	Leg	Hips

Keep a MEASUREMENT CHART like this in your journal.

▪ Look at your body.

☑ Snap a picture of your body. Actually, snap several. Use your phone or iPad or a DSLR and snap your body from the front, sides, and back. Wear something form-fitting or revealing like workout clothes, a swimsuit, or under garments. Natural daytime lighting will give you a fair picture. Keep your photos in your journal or POST THEM alongside **your posted** written and visual goals (including the magazine clippings that represent your desired body and experience).

☑ Look at yourself in a full-body mirror. Do it every day. Research shows those who look at their goals every day are more likely to accomplish them because the

goals stay at front of mind. Your body is your
meaningful goal.

Whenever I create art with either clay, paints, or jewelry,
I first conceive a mental image of what I intend to see or
feel. I apply colors, shapes, and textures, periodically
stepping away to observe my progress. I add detail to
deepen and clarify my creation.

Master bakers collect their ingredients, mix the dry and
wet ones in their separate bowls, fold the ingredients
together, then taste to determine what's needed and
what's in excess. A master violinist writes a first
composition, listens, adds harmonies, cuts extraneous
notes, and refines the intensity with accents, volume, and
tonality. Like artists, bakers, and music makers, spend
time looking, tweaking, and connecting with your piece
of art, you. Look at your body. Communicate with your
body.

UNDRAPE YOUR MASTERPIECE

One reason bodyweight swells during the winter months
is because the body gets buried under layers of down,
wool, and flannel. It's easy to disconnect from a body
you don't see regularly.

If you're advance-scheduling your workouts, you're most likely at the gym looking at your "goal" in a large mirror often. Good job. Which leads to another observation: baggy gym clothes are hiding your results from becoming your new normal.

IS THIS YOU?

You're in the front row of an exercise class doing your jumping jacks and push-ups. You've lost 15 lbs this year. You can comfortably fit into a size medium tank top, yet you're still wearing the triple large t-shirt and slouchy sweats you wore last year. First of all, why are you hiding under clothes large enough to fit you and three kids? Why are you wearing clothes that don't fit you anymore? If you keep sending the message to your brain that *triple large is what I wear* or *I don't want to see my body because I still don't like it*, your habit of mind will match your body. This baggy habit can negatively result in gaining some of the weight back to match your belief about yourself.

As your clothes become baggier, they'll reflect who you were, not who you are now. Dress in clothes that fit who you've become, especially during your workouts.

- Your zipper ain't gonna lie.

I own a pair of lovely skinny jeans. Whenever I wear those black jeans I know if I've had too many cheat brownies in a week. When that zipper leaves teeth marks in my belly, I immediately launch a course-correction and re-vision my meaningful goals.

First of all following my initial weight loss, it took 10 years to muster enough nerve to buy a pair of jeans. During my early twenties when I hid my leg and belly fat behind untucked shirts and hippy-styled skirts, I vowed I'd never wear jeans. I'd gotten traumatized in a JCPenney dressing room at the day I swore jeans away. With four pairs on the floor and two more to try-on, all sized between 9-12, I'd failed to find a pair that fit.My shape was odd. Broad shoulders. Small waist with a little pooch. The circumference of my legs could fool a football coach if he didn't see the face that belonged to them. Jeans that fit my thick legs needed a rope to fasten the huge waist. Trying on jeans was a futile effort, so I never wore them.

I returned to jeans on a Saturday in the winter of 2007. Even though I'd been working as a trainer for years by then, and even though I'd won two bodybuilding shows

by then, I was still afraid of denim. My PROGRAM had
kept reminding me that *I have big, fat legs.*

I bravely selected several pairs of jeans to try—sizes
10,12, and 14. The legs fit in the size 10 pair, thanks to
spandex in the denim. The waist was way too big, of
course.

I didn't give up. I hunted two more pairs, an 8 and a 6,
prompted by the sales lady who thought I wore a 6
anyway. The size 6 jeans went over my legs and zipped.
In shock, I checked the size on the tag inside the jeans.
They fit my butt perfectly. I did a solo boogie in that
dressing room then bought two pairs in size 6.

Seeing myself in those jeans, smashed my old
PROGRAM. You will change your PROGRAM, too. When
you courageously place the 8 healthy habits of **The RiT**
in motion, your mind and body will transform.

You might feel compelled to save those baggy Levis you
bought in college. You've had them for 8 years, two
boyfriends, and an unforgettable trip to St. Louis. You
might think to stash 'em under your bed in a plastic
storage tub, saved for the day when... maybe... just in
case... in case you gain the weight back.

Don't save 'em.

If you're apprehensive about getting rid of the "old you"
clothes, give 'em a good-bye ceremony. Play music.
Frank Sinatra. Jay-Z. Baroque concertos. Cut those oversized tees and baggy sweats into rags. I give you
permission.

Get rid of the "old you" clothes. Get rid of everything that
doesn't fit you anymore. Wear clothes that fit you. Look
in the mirror. See how far you've progressed. Tell
yourself you've progressed.

These suggestions for gauging whether you're
succeeding with your fat-loss are unconventional
methods, I agree. I suggest these simple methods
because they'll motivate you more often than a scale.

**These suggestions will positively influence the way you
see yourself and the way you feel.**

- The result of your doctor's report is a reliable
record of your health and fitness.

Your doctor can generally clear you to begin a specific
exercise and healthy food program.

Your blood work and/or cardiograph report will provide
an efficient report of your health. Your doctor can assist
by advising whether there are contraindicated exercises
(not appropriate for your body at the time) and if there
are exercises that are recommended for your needs.
Get a *physical check-up* every year at minimum. Create
a folder of your doctor's reports so you can compare
your past with your present health.

FIND A TRIBE THAT ALIGNS WITH YOUR VIBE

So it goes that you must uphold your boundaries around your sacred workout schedule. Live your quality decision to be healthy and fit. Of course you expect your loved ones and friends to cheer you through your evolution. Maybe they will. It would be ideal. But they might not.

Some OPOs aren't ready or willing to uproot their old beliefs, so they might not be ready to see you dump yours either. However, you need to have someone who supports you in your camp.

You've gotta find someone who fervently supports your agenda and your opinion; someone who can feed you inspiration.

You will be more successful sustaining your fat loss when you have company. You need support. Arnold Schwarzenegger had a trainer. Serena Williams had a coach. Don't go it alone. Find a tribe that aligns with your vibe.

• • •

If you want to go fast, go alone.

If you want to go far, go together.

An African proverb

Do you remember Elliot and Anna from my fat-loss journey? Well, years after I moved away from my soothsayer, Elliot, and my aerobic chief, Anna, I met Crystal. She was my first aerobic teacher in New York City who eventually become my boss. Goss was a peer trainer who coached me to become stronger than I'd ever been. They held me to high standards and pushed my boundaries to reach farther than what I thought was possible. I gathered workout buddies along my path like Norma and Cecilia, two fierce lifters who became supportive peers in the weight room. I have always kept magazine clippings and saved videos from a crew of torchbearers including Jackie Joyner Kersey, Serena Williams, and Brandon Carter.

Several peer fitness instructors and many of my students have become my tribe of support pushing me to physical excellence.

Anchor your tent with support from one or all of these relationships: a teacher, a trainer, or a friend.

A teacher.
A teacher is someone whose message fans your flame—someone who knows you, sees your skills, and inspires you to express your full potential.
A trainer.
A trainer sets the compass to keep you on-course toward your meaningful goals—someone who crafts a plan that holds you to a high standard of behavior and guides you to visualize and speak yourself into your meaningful goal.

A friend. A buddy.
A workout partner who challenges you as well as celebrates results with you—the two or group of you can tick off your progress points as you work toward your meaningful goals together.

Make certain your teacher, trainer, and/or friend raises a set of expectations that push past your previous limitations. Make sure your teacher, trainer, or friend helps you safely execute the 8 habits of health and fitness. They must support your "new normal" and celebrate your wins.

ALL YOU NEED IS...

You don't have to accept it, if it's not love.

This is your message especially if you're either new to following an exercise and health plan or if you haven't been able to sustain your fat-loss journey.

In the summer of 2000, I trained for a bodybuilding show. I knew the decision would come as a shock to many of my peers. I'd spent twenty years singing and dancing on stages around the country. When I became a personal trainer in 1997, my tribe of friends and family couldn't conceive of me as an *athlete.* To them, I was a song-writer and poet and didn't fit the profile of a heavy lifter or a personal trainer.

I secretly prepared for my first bodybuilding show in 1999. Only a couple clients and three fellow trainers knew what I was planning. Mind you, I was training like a wild woman, first gaining muscle all winter, then leaning-out by April. My abs were totally ripped. My back was a muscle anatomy chart. I was doing chin ups, an exercise women didn't readily do in my gym. I was napping on breaks between clients. These are all the things bodybuilders do, yet no one asked me why I was doing them. I guess they thought I was preparing for the beach season.

Most of the trainers from my health club came to see me win my first bodybuilding show. I hadn't told them about the contest until the week of the show.

Why did I keep my show a secret? I didn't want input. I feared most of my community would have been my OPOs. I was correct about that.

I announced my second show which was nine weeks later. Weekly I received unsolicited advice and opinions from other trainers. Even gym members thought to comment with their opinions about I should or shouldn't do. Just as I'd expected. OPOs interject their feedback when it's not warranted and when they have no experience with the sport of bodybuilding. Don't let OPOs distract you.

You see, before I did my first show, I was terrified— absolutely, terrified. Unsure if I'd be able to maintain my training regimen, afraid I wouldn't be able to burn the cellulite from my legs, needing to learn know how to pose properly, I honestly didn't know what my body would be able to do. The challenge of setting new habits of mind and heart despite my fears consumed my energy. I didn't need unsolicited questions and opinions to rattle my focus.

I only told people I knew for sure would affirm my personal lovetruths and meaningful feeling goals. I chose people who supported the vision I had for myself or better. I chose to tell people who would not distract me, but inspire me. Their intention matched mine.

To this day, when I aim to manifest something that scares me, even a little, I ONLY tell the people who will encourage my vision. **No OPOs of OPAs are allowed in my head.**

There are people in your world who **will definitely** cheer you on. Find them. Do your best not to let your power get diffused by the negative opinions, lack of belief, and discouragement from folks who are more scared than you. Remain silent around the doubters. What they share with you will be debilitating. Surround yourself with a tribe of warriors.

• • •

You don't need everybody, but you do need somebody.
Michelle Bernard

MAKE PEACE WITH TIME

No matter how excited you become to hurry toward your goals, remain steady. Slow, steady progress leads to sustainable results. The bathroom scale will display your efforts best it can, but the other four methods for measuring fat-loss and health are more reliable.

Remain diligent. It takes time and consistency to strengthen your muscles and acclimate your body to shorter, intense cardio and strength training workouts. Within 6 months to a year you'll be able to handle higher levels of intensity in shorter workout sessions.

When you first begin *The RiTual* you'll see immediate results. Between weeks 8 and 12, your results might halt. You'll wonder why your body's not changing anymore. Sometimes a plateau means you're body's reached a maintenance phase and you need to raise your workout intensity for more changes to occur. Fat-loss plateaus are common and they'll come around more than once.

Most women have a **set-point weight range,** fluctuating weight between 2-3 pounds. But you may have noticed the challenge of losing weight happens when you hit set-point weight range.

Homeostasis is the body's way of resisting radical change. It accounts for the plateau and the challenge of losing weight beyond your set-point weight range.

Consistent exercise with a gradual increase in intensity along with a healthy fuel plan will alter your body composition and lower your set-point weight range. Don't let a plateau stop you. Keep going.

There's another set-point that isn't discussed much, but if you don't acknowledge it, it can thwart your progress. **You have a mental set-point that can challenge your belief about what you can accept for yourself.**

The mental set-point revs up when you experience positive results.

Zoey dried the sweat from her forehead, wrapped herself in a towel, and stepped out of the steam room. Zoey hadn't weighed herself in three months. Before her shower, she stepped on it. 142 pounds.
Zoey ate her regular post-workout meal in the parking lot: a small bowl of lentils with pickled cabbage, avocado, and quinoa. On the drive home, she stopped for frozen yogurt but changed her mind and ordered three scoops of coffee ice cream.

The next day, Zoey was overcome by the smell of her mother's homemade lasagna. She helped herself to three heaping squares. Zoey took a 30-minute walk with her sister after dinner.

*The next day, Zoey walked on the track in the university gym instead going to her regular kickboxing class. Afterward she planted herself at the burger pub on campus to study. She ordered a cheddar cheese burger with sweet potato fries, a meal she hadn't ordered in over 6 months. Zoey became sleepy and left the pub after an hour after eating. She didn't know why she was tired or why she craved fattening foods day after day. She was battling the crazings. Immediately she journaled her feelings. She decided to return to practicing the 8 habits of **The RiT**.*

That evening she made a delicious lean and green meal.

Zoey had successfully practiced **The RiT** for 6 consistent months. What made her snap into the crazings?

Zoey was challenged by her weight-loss accomplishment. Over-eating was the unconscious way she distanced herself her new normal weight of 142 pounds. She hadn't weighed 142 pounds since her first year of high school and she felt uncomfortable with the result. **Zoey was afraid she wouldn't be able to maintain her new normal weight.** Zoey "craved" a way to relieve the pressure. Her fear made her hungry to return to a weight she could accept.

You deserve health and happiness, regardless of your past, regardless of your genes, and regardless of what anybody else thinks. Practice your lovetruth visualization to see yourself in a new way. Become the way your heart has defined you, not the world, not your past, not limitation, and not your fear.

SQUIRREL!

You're putting your groceries in the fridge, a stock of fresh vegetables for the week. You feel good about your grocery choices until you check your Facebook feed. Two "friends" from high school (you weren't friends with in high school) have posted a video about how they lost 20 pounds in 12 days on a bacon and beef jerky diet. SQUIRREL.

A smiling redhead with no fat anywhere has posted a video of the purple contraption she uses to do 1000 crunches a day.
SQUIRREL.

Your buddy from work is taking six pink pills with a special breakfast flatbread and has lost 28 pounds this month...
SQUIRREL.

Fat-defying contraptions and miracle pills are big business. The lordships of pop-up ads promote a new weight-loss thingy every new moon. It can be tempting to rubber neck these miracles because, for rascal's sake, you've willing to try anything to look photoshopped in reality.

Don't get vaporized into the black hole of *I could lose weight faster without working out, without giving up fast food, with my eyes totally closed, by eating whenever and whatever I want.*

Too many fitness and diet programs swirling in your head at once will distract you from making progress.

Stay focused. Slick marketing promising that *you can do nothing and still lose* fat is never true.

It's a SQUIRREL you will never catch, Fido. Focus—on one program—at a time. Focus on one program that is holistic and sustainable as a lifestyle. Because if it isn't sustainable, you won't live healthy beyond a few hungry weeks.

(If you've seen the animated movie *UP!* you understand the SQUIRREL reference. If you haven't, SQUIRREL means distraction.)

The next thing I'm about to tell you might make you cry. It could make you so angry about reading this far that you slam the remaining pages of this book onto your innocent thumb. Or maybe you'll swallow hard and say, *Bring it, Michelle. I'm ready for anything.*

You aren't going to lose fat, get fit, and sustain a healthy lifestyle by traveling an "easy" road.

Here's why.

From this day on you're **not** going to be able to do what everybody else is doing. You'll be more conscious than you were before. You'll have to be mindful about putting away old habits and picking up new healthier habits. You'll have to automate some of your daily decisions to avoid life's temptations. Do you remember when I discussed this in the beginning of this book?

You know what? I've transformed from a hopeless, pudgy non-believer who was sure **exercise would NOT work for me**, into a fit, healthy, aware, and gloriously disciplined being. Yet, each and every week I must STILL remind myself, *You can do this, Michelle. You are worth it, Michelle.*

It's enticing to think about eating whatever I want, skipping workouts, bingeing on cookie dough while watching season 7 of RuPaul's Drag Race (again).

I still have wandering eyes for a brownie or three. But once I rein in my imagination from flirting with the fudge, I can regain a glimpse of my meaningful vision. I remember what matters. I'd rather feel like a super queen of the world, than pissed because nothing in my closet zips (the way I used to feel). I can wait for my cheat brownie, anyway.

Even though I love to exercise now, I'm challenged when I'm scheduled to workout alone. I still might start a conversation with myself to try and get out of it. But after 5 minutes of jumping on my trampoline to DIM ALL THE LIGHTS, I feel like a champ again. I'm proud of myself again. I admire my grit again. I believe in my vision once more.

I think you might be like me. You have a voice inside that course-corrects your impulses, that supports your vision. Like me, you have a voice that will question, *Why am I choosing two bowls of cereal before bed? Why am I skipping spinning class to watch DEXTER reruns?*

That voice inside is not scolding. She is the voice of your visionary. That voice is your hope. It's your heart. It'll never leave you even if you try to hush it, even if you go against it.

Align with that voice inside, your visionary voice, your heart. You will find your freedom. I know you will. Trust yourself.

You are special enough, worthy enough, and visionary enough to succeed at your fitness and wellness goals. Trust my voice, too.

Transform your mind, body and your life
with healthy **h.a.b.i.t.s**

::

harness your creative mind
abandon your barriers,
bring a desired vision and feeling into your body,
initiate a series of behaviors that align with your vision
and you will

transform your body, your mind,

and your life.

Though this process isn't easy-peasy, fast and furious, or sweet and skippy every day; it is, for sure, the best stuff in town.

Start living healthy.

Keep living healthy.

Live, my love.

Only from the heart can

you touch the sky

RUMI

The benefits of consistently living the 8 healthy habits of
The RiTual

::

[hear the crowd roar with applause as you read the list]

Lower stress

Lower body fat

Increased muscle tone

Reduced cravings and fewer desires to binge

Conscious and creative eating

Increased flexibility and strength

Quality rest

Body awareness

Self confidence

Enhanced mood

Self-awareness

PART FIVE

YOUR HAPPY PLACE

• • •

Our culture has a sphincter over having too much fun.
Dr. Christiane Northrup,
author of the iconic Women's Bodies, Women's Wisdom
and Goddesses Never Age

I've added a ninth habit. This one's responsible for most of your happiness. Perhaps this ninth habit is why centenarians in The Blue Zones practice live long, healthy lives.

Learning about the lifestyle of people living in The Blue Zones has regulated my blood pressure. The Blue Zones represent several small communities around the world where the people live longer (and collectively happier) than other areas. Blue Zone communities reside in Ikaria, Greece; Sardinia, Italy; Nicoya, Costa Rica; Okinawa, Japan; and one city in Loma Linda, California.

The people in The Blue Zones don't exclusively eat low-fat foods. They don't swipe gym cards 4–6 days a week. They don't need to **advance-schedule** a **Body of Exercise** nor do they eat every 4 hours. In Dan Buettner's book, The Blue Zones, he examines the health practices of the communities.

For instance, more than 10% of the population in Ikaria, Greece is over 100 years old with the women living up to 112 years old, many have never visited a hospital. Many in this community rarely experience depression or disease.

The people of Ikaria, Greece grow their own food and eat from the sea. Their daily exercise consists of planting and gathering the food grown over hilly landscapes. It's common to share group meals with music, dancing, and laughing. A couple glasses of freshly harvested red wine is usually served.

They live slower paced, community-focused lives. Stress is low, if present at all. They enjoy their work. Retirement is uncommon. And, they nap.

They enjoy nature and POSSIBILITY thinking. They enjoy being alive. The ninth habit I offer you is: **Enjoy your life.** Connect with people and experiences that bring you joy. The ninth habit is **experience joy.**

What brings you pleasure? What makes you laugh? What makes your eyes light up and come alive?

Recall the HeartMath research in habit #2. When you participate in activities, experiences, and engage in thoughts and feelings that bring you joy, your bodily and mental improves.

MAGIC LIGHT

As a kid in Iowa, I thought lightening bugs were most magical. Their flickering light is caused by **nitric oxide.** Your body produces your own nitric oxide when you belly-laugh. You also get a big dose of this magic flickering during meditations and during orgasms.

Nitric oxide lowers your blood pressure. It improves circulation so nutrients can support your organs. It reduces inflammation, improves your immune response, and promotes better sleep. Are you laughing, having an orgasm, or meditating regularly?

You can also increase nitric oxide by exercising and by eating. Choose walnuts, spinach, brown rice, cranberries, salmon, and kale.

Here's the yuck news. Your body produces less nitric oxide if you smoke, when you abstain from exercise, if you're obese, and when you don't manage your stress overload. Once your nitric oxide production decreases, it's hard to rev it up again.

Eek! There's more. Negative thinking lowers your nitric oxide. If you're chronically angsty, irritated, and pissed or if you experience prolonged grief, your magic light goes out.

Just because someone exercises, doesn't mean they are producing the magic. Imagine the grinch runner. I've seen this kind of runner in Central Park hunched over in pain as they go. Their shoulders are tense, with angry eyes dreading each stride. The grinch runner has waged a war with the fat and hates running as much as they hate their body. The grinch runner blames life for their inner dissatisfaction.

Then there's the red-eyed aerobic student. This one never smiles during class. This one has come to punish their body. They want the workout to hurt because they're also mad at the fat.

And have you met the serial dieter? This one tries every diet program. Agitated, she snaps off the lid to eat her lettuce and lemons. Her co-worker's spicy burrito hits her nostril. She explains, ad nauseam, that she can't eat burritos and that she'll probably get fat just smelling it. She's always complaining about what she can't eat and why. People avoid taking their lunch break when they see her in the cafeteria.

An angry pursuit for perfection. Swallowing resentment for lunch. The absence of joy within a healthy lifestyle plan doesn't make any sense.

THE HAPPY RETURN

Instead of focusing on what you don't have, value the skills, abilities, and parts of your body you do have. Dream of what's possible. Move toward it in body and mind. Fall in love with your vision. Fall in love with this healthy journey.

CAMP OUT

PRACTICE THE HABIT

Habit #9 <u>Live a joyful life. Notice what makes you grateful. Laugh.</u>

Spend your life with folks that light you up. Spend time in nature. Explore your creativity or start a hobby. Pet an animal, touch someone or let yourself be touched, pray or dance your prayer. Laugh. Often.

Make a list of experiences and activities that bring you joy and make you laugh.

Like ➠ reading inspirational texts, singing, walking in the park, bathing in salts and aroma, knitting, painting, watching comedies, sewing, massage, game night with friends, masturbation, scrapbooking, making love, dancing, laughing, gardening, going to the theatre or a concert, playing board games with others, putting a puzzle together, attending a book club, expressing yourself fully...

1.

2.

3.

4.

5.

6.

7.

Can you advance-schedule 1-2 pleasurable activities this month (besides exercise)?

I will____

on (date or day)_________________________________.

I will____

on (date or day)_________________________________.

Contemplate what you love about your life. Write about this in your journal. Sit with this love during your mental massage.

LEAN HAPPY HEALTHY YOU Journal

What have been your biggest obstacles while practicing the 8 healthy habits of The RiT?

What have been your biggest breakthroughs while practicing the 8 healthy habits of The RiT?

What new experiences have you been exposed to because of your healthy lifestyle practice?

In what ways do you feel more confident since you've begun practicing The RiT?

Who is supporting you to live healthy?

Are you supporting another person to live healthier?

Write some of the compliments you've received since beginning your healthy lifestyle.

How do these compliments make you feel?

The ~~end~~ beginning.

• • •

Your imagination can penetrate your life.

Michelle Bernard

ABOUT THE AUTHOR

Michelle Bernard, MS Ed, is a wellness educator, author, and artist.

Born in Iowa, she's lived in the cities of her dreams, Chicago, Los Angeles, Osaka, Japan, and Manhattan; performing as a singer and poet as well as teaching fitness and yoga programs to children, adults, and seniors.

She was awarded a New York City Teaching Fellowship for her Master's degree in Education. She established the Theatre Arts department at 754X, a high school for students with special needs in the Bronx.

She also developed the curriculum for Creative Movement for Enlightened Minds and Stand in Your Light, her yoga and drama youth programs, respectively, for CUNY in the Heights in Manhattan.

Her devotional yoga offering at Amsterdam Day Program in Manhattan used chair dancing, Hatha yoga, and active imagination to help seniors breathe deeper, move with joy, and recall satisfying memories.

Michelle currently supports humans who think it's groovy to be strong, spirited, and wild with J.A.M. Sessions (Journal Art & Movement) and WiLD journaling programs.

Michelle plays the tennis channel all day, soaks in salt baths at night, and adores stepping out into sunny Mondays (which she does weekly since moving to Florida in 2019).

When Michelle isn't sculpting bodies or painting curiosities, you can find her in a corner cafe with her journal. Meet her there. Tell her your stories over a coffee—or seven.

Making muscles, meaning, and a strong cup of coffee are most fulfilling.

Special thanks to my clients and to the students from my exercise classes for their ongoing support while writing this book.

You complete me,
Michelle Bernard

Michelle Bernard, MS Ed is a Wellness Educator & Artist. She's the creator of J.A.M. Sessions, JOURNAL | ART | MOVEMENT, workshops for self-liberation through fitness, Hatha yoga, WiLD journaling, and Intentional Creativity painting.

Catch her vibe at
liveaboveordinary.teachable.com

REFERENCES AND LINKS

Referenced Internet

http://www.who.int/mediacentre/factsheets/fs311/en/

http://stateofobesity.org/obesity-rates-trends-overview/

https://www.washingtonpost.com/news/to-your-health/wp/2015/06/22/americas-getting-even-fatter-startling-growth-in-obesity-over-past-20-years/

http://consumer.healthday.com/encyclopedia/diabetes-13/misc-diabetes-news-181/type-2-diabetes-and-kids-the-growing-epidemic-644152.html

http://www.gallup.com/poll/170264/adult-obesity-rate.aspx

http://www.health.harvard.edu/blog/artificial-sweeteners-sugar-free-but-at-what-cost-201207165030

http://www.stress.org/stress-effects/

https://sleepfoundation.org/sleep-topics/napping

http://theweightofthenation.hbo.com/themes/what-is-obesity

http://ajcn.nutrition.org/content/94/2/601.abstract?sid=c3d63130-3cc4-47e1-9441-ac56483087f1

https://umm.edu/health/medical/altmed/herb/green-tea

http://www.helpguide.org/articles/sleep/how-much-sleep-do-you-need.htm

http://adrenalfatiguesolution.com/stress-immune-system/

http://www.heartmathinstitute.com

http://www.zazenlife.com

http://www.hayhouseradio.com

Referenced Books

Each book offers an education from the university of fulfillment.
These books will change the way you experience your life and
your body.

Breaking the Habit of Being Yourself, Dr. Joe Dispenza

Power vs Force, Dr. David Hawkins

The Motivation Manifesto, Brendon Burchard

The Powermind System - Twelve lessons on the Psychology of
Success, Michael Monroe Kiefer

The Power of Habit, Dr. Charles Duhigg

Heart Intelligence, Doc Childre, Deborah Rozman, Rollin
McCraty, Howard Martin of HeartMath Institute

Goddesses Never Age, Dr. Christiane Northrup

Wishes Fulfilled, Dr. Wayne Dyer

"What the Bleep Do You Know?"

This scientific docu-movie explores Masuro Emoto's water experiment as well as how we create potentials with our powerful thoughts.

ESTIMATE YOUR HEART RATE

Estimate your workout intensity with this **perceived exertion** chart. Gauge your cardio intensity by noticing how you feel.

Use this fun guideline to gauge your *perceived level of exertion* during your 20–60 minute cardio workout.

Level of *perceived exertion* between 1 – 10.

You're working out at level...

::

1 = **SNORE.** Similar to sleeping.
You're yawning and dozing off even though your arms and feet are moving.

2 = **BORED**. Like walking a bored dog through the park—while wearing stilettos—you, not the dog.

4 = **DRY.** If you can say, *I never sweat when I workout.* This is probably why.

6 = **ALMOST.** Even though your voice is loud and somewhat breathy, you're able to chat on your cellphone.
Listen, working out while talking on the phone shouldn't be happening.
Hang up. Your caller can wait 45 minutes.
Plus, you're about to rise into the perfect breathing zone.

8-9 = POWER. This is it! You would prefer not to talk at all at this pace. Instead, you're focusing on your alignment while moving through a full range of motion.

You feel powerful.

This is the workout intensity that will transform your body, the desirable aerobic breathing pace.

10 = **BURST.** You're unable to catch the 4th, 5th, or 6th breath after 3 minutes at this breathing pace.

Your chest might hurt at this heart rate.

You need to slowdown but not slow enough to walk your bored dog in stilettos.

Try to get back to intensity **8—POWER.**

UNBREAKABLE?

MAKE IT, THEN BREAK IT

You're gonna break the habits of *The RiT—sort of...*

After you've implemented *The RiTual* for 9 consecutive months and after experiencing significant fat-loss, lean muscle gain, stronger bones, and more confidence, I want you to break the habits of *The RiT*—some of it.

Shatter two of the habits: your schedule and your fuel.

For ONE week:

1. Break your **workout schedule.** Reduce it from 4-6 days a week to as little as **1-2 workouts for ONE week ONLY.** (Habit #4)
2. Break your **fuel cycle from 4 hour intervals to 5-6 hour intervals daily for ONE week ONLY.** (Habit #6)

After you've been practicing *The RiTual* **for 9 consecutive months,** break these two habits for **ONE WEEK ONLY.**

This will fit perfectly into your life if you have a vacation planned to say, Greece, and there's no exercise facility in your hotel. To be honest, I have found it difficult to break the workout portion of *The RiT*. I worked out 4 times during my first week in Greece. I substituted other physical activities like walking and hiking during my second week. I was in Mykonos, Greece, not Ikaria with the centenarians, but the frequent walks from the hotel into town coupled with the fresh local foods and sea foods, made it an ideal week to break *The RiT*.

A **one week departure** from these two habits won't give you cause to worry about gaining the weight back. That is, if you keep eating from your desirable grocery list with the *eat with your hands* portions. Don't fret if you mysteriously gain 1-2 pounds on a scale. Likely, it's just water weight because you're not sweating the way you would be if you were working out 5 times a week. You will lose that water when you return to your sweaty workout schedule.

Your body needs this rest for muscle and joint recovery. One week of rest and recovery can prevent over-use injuries. Feel free to practice light FLEXIBILITY and/or RELAXATION training during your break week.
Your muscles may have endured low-grade pulls and strains. Resting your muscles for one week lets the tissues heal and regain strength. Your connective tissue,

especially your knee joints, elbows, and shoulders, need
a respite from high-intensity and heavy/repetitive weight-
bearing movements.

The break will help you overcome a fat-loss plateau.
When you return to advance-scheduling 4-6 workouts,
you're likely to feel so strong and refreshed. You'll be
able to push your intensity up a notch. Within a couple
weeks following your return to *The RiT,* you'll drop
another pound automatically, plus you'll flush water
weight you might have gained. Every time you increase
your strength and workout intensity, you create a fat-loss
opportunity.

So, break habits #4 and #6 (the number of workouts
and fuel intervals) from *The RiTual* for ONE week.

<u>Every 6 months thereafter,</u>
Break *The RiT* for one week.

When you return to *The RiT*, EAT CLEAN for 2 weeks
(refer to Habit #6 to review fuel), then return to fueling
as noted in the 8 healthy habits of *The RiT.*

For now, continue to listen to the voice in your heart.
It will remind you what matters every day. You do.

Your health does.
You're worth it.

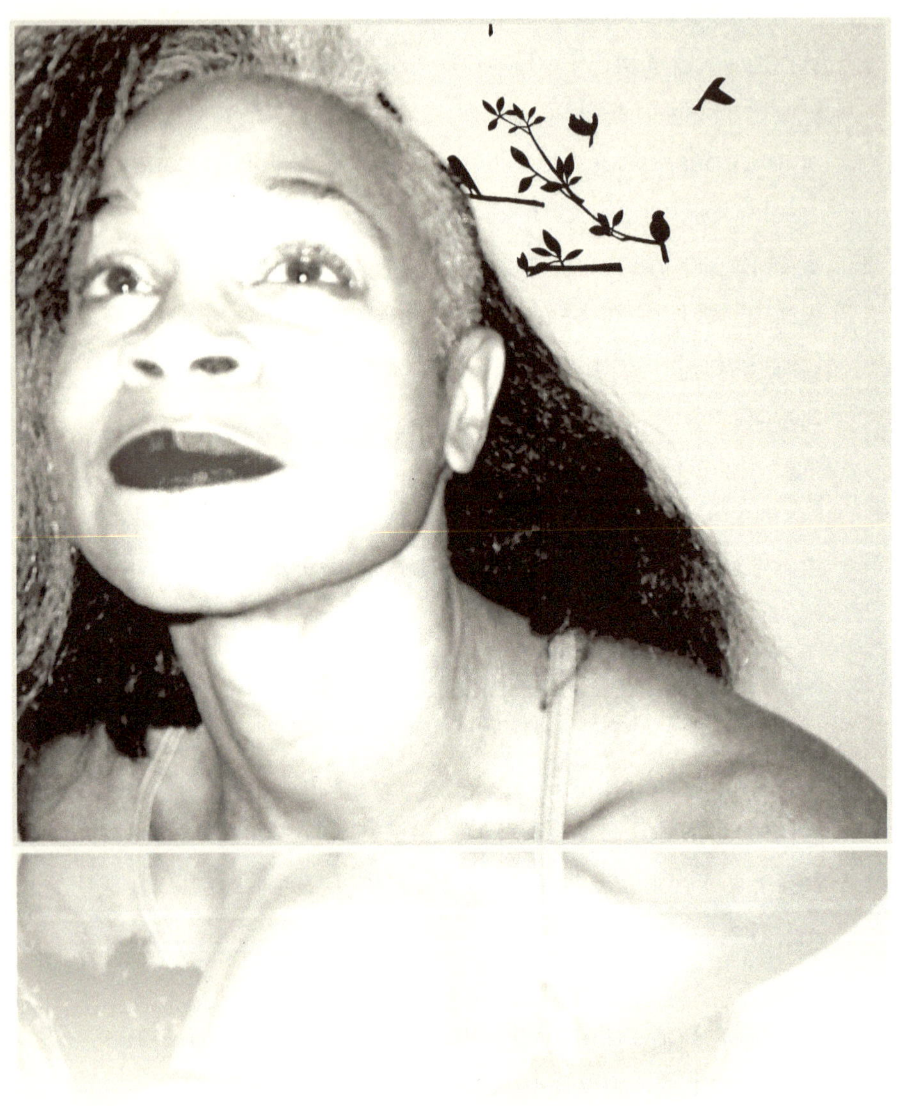

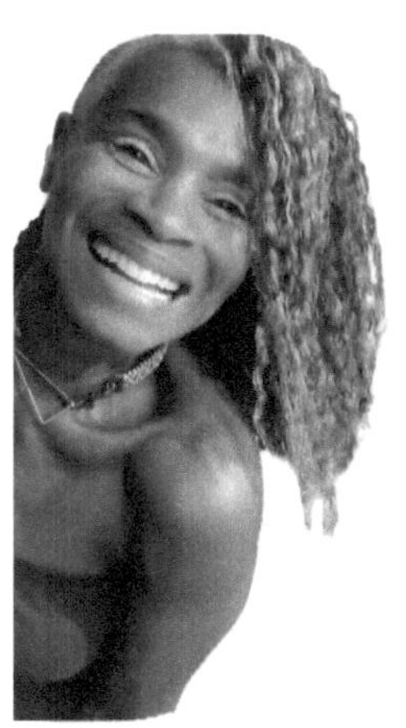

MY FAVORITE THINGS

Here are few of my favorite things

the TRX—suspension training exercise equipment
the stability ball—balance training exercise equipment
the foam roller—muscle recovery equipment
dumbbells—of course
trampoline—yippie

Coconut Oil for hair and skin and cooking, oh my

the VitaMixer

chalkboard paint

✳

See More
www.kit.co/michellebernard

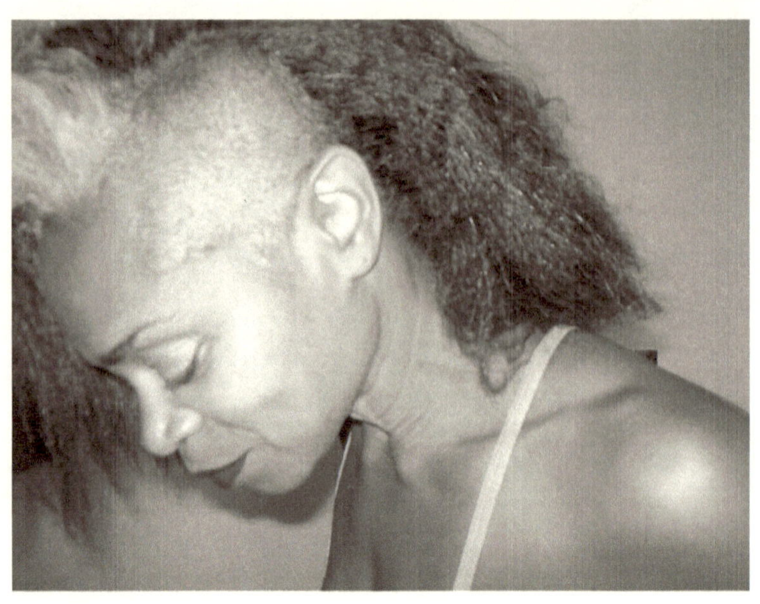

Journal | Art | Movement

The Live Above Ordinary Oasis, for humans who believe
it's groovy to be strong, spirited, and wild.

liveaboveordinary.teachable.com

studiomichellebernard.com

Michelle Bernard's BOOKS and JOURNALS

PAPER COACH, a wellness journal & log

WHATEVER | a journal for the stuff I think – for tweens & teens

beyond words—finding fulfillment between the lines

the black coffee journal series

Journaling Card Decks

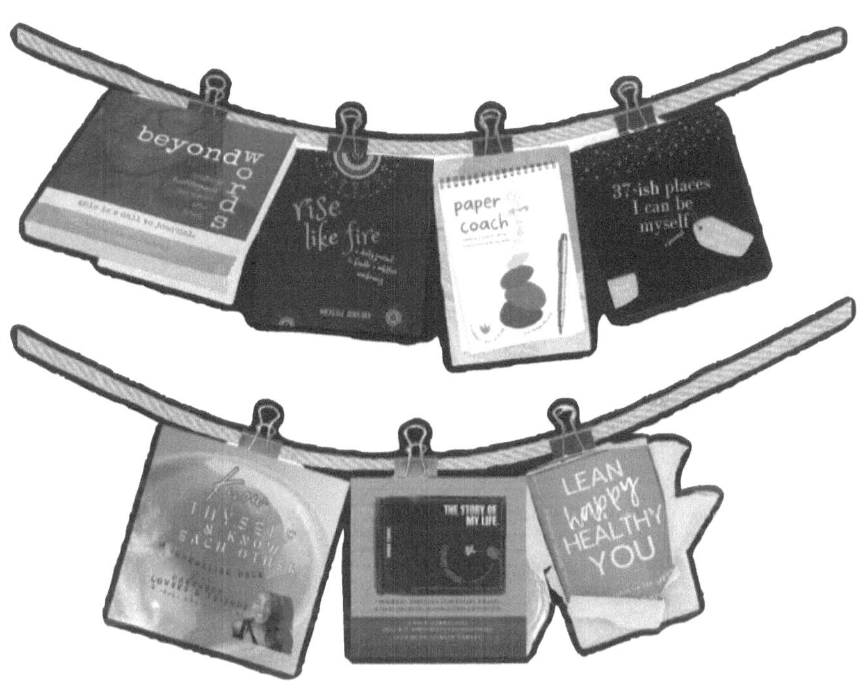

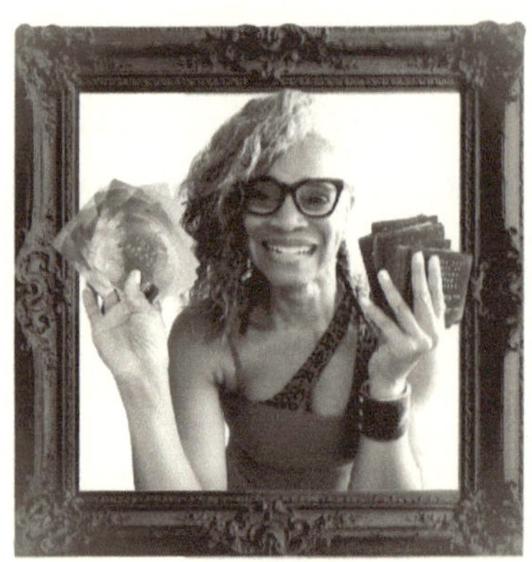

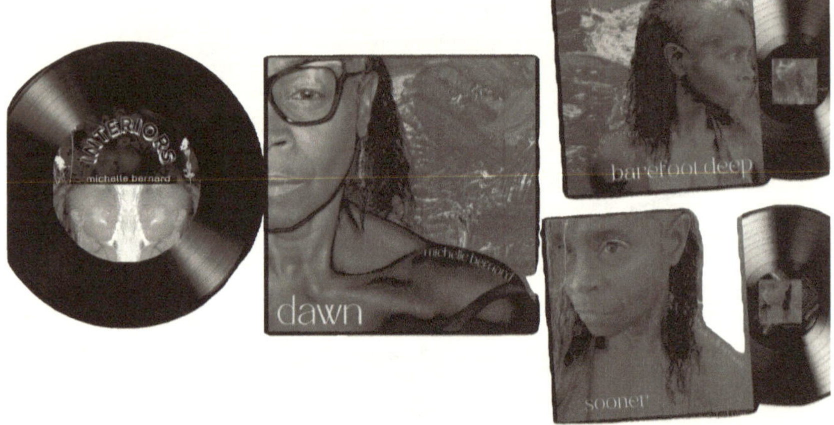

Michelle Bernard's Music & Art

Albums: **INTERIORS, DAWN, BAREFOOT DEEP, SOONER**

Streaming everywhere

studiomichellebernard.com

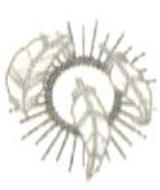